STEMI

3-Minute Diagnosis, 90-Minute Reperfusion
Saving Time, Saves Lives

A Primer of STEMI EKGs for Early Cath Lab Activation.

Marco Mercader, MD, FACC, FHRS
Associate Professor
Division of Cardiology and Cardiac Electrophysiology
Medical Faculty Associates
The George Washington University

P. Jacob Varghese, MD, FRCP, FACC
Director of the Coronary Care Unit
Professor Emeritus of Medicine and Pediatrics
Medical Faculty Associates
The George Washington University

Mortada A. Shams, MD
Resident Physician
Division of Internal Medicine
The George Washington University Hospital

Alexander E. Sullivan, BSc
Medical Student
The George Washington School of Medicine and Health Sciences

Abudureyimu Shajidan, MD
Visiting Scholar
Xinjiang Medical University, Xinjiang, China

Bassel Hassouna, MD
Cardiology Fellow
Division of Cardiology
The George Washington University Hospital

Vimala V. Jayanthi, MD, FACP
Assistant Professor of Medicine
Medical Faculty Associates
The George Washington University

Table of Contents

Preface

3-Minute Diagnosis, 90-Minute Reperfusion
Saving Time, Saves Lives

In the last 10 years, cardiovascular mortality has dropped by 30 percent. This is the result of various innovations in preventive cardiology, diagnostic testing, and treatment modalities. None affected the outcome of myocardial infarction more than the 90-minute reperfusion strategy, the so-called "DOOR to Balloon Time". This approach has resulted in a 5 percent, 30-day mortality rate for an acute myocardial infarction.

To achieve this result, every caregiver of an acute ST elevation myocardial infarction (STEMI) patient – the medical student, resident physician, cardiology fellow, ER physician, attending, and first responder – should be proficient in diagnosing a STEMI in the EKG, so that they can activate the cath lab. This book is designed to achieve that purpose.

This book has three sections. The first section illustrates the classical EKG changes of the various types of STEMI. The second section shows the equivalent STEMI presentations. The third section shows EKGs that mimic a STEMI. The best way to use this book is to take a pre-test, study the material and then take a post-test. In the post-test, our aim is for the participant to achieve the accuracy of cath lab activation of 95 percent. With that knowledge one can implement a 3-minute diagnosis and a 90-minute reperfusion strategy and thereby achieving a 30-day mortality in acute myocardial infarction of 5 percent.

This book is a result of the collaborative work of medical students, residents, cardiology fellows, attendings and electrophysiologists.

P. Jacob Varghese, M.D, F.R.C.P, F.A.C.C
Professor Emeritus of Medicine and Pediatrics
Director of the Coronary Care Unit
The George Washington University
Washington D.C.

How to Use this Book

This is a self study guide comprised of 24 cases seen at George Washington University Hospital. We provide the presenting EKGs with their corresponding coronary angiogram, echocardiogram or CT-angiogram images, obtained during management.

A brief introductory segment is followed by a case-by-case analysis of important, evidence-based EKG findings in STEMIs, STEMI-equivalents, and STEMI-mimics. The goal is to improve STEMI recognition skills, thereby improving cath lab activation accuracy to help achieve a 90-minute reperfusion strategy.

After reading the introduction, go through the cases. Read each EKG in a systematic fashion. Consider the context of the clinical history provided and interpret the EKG, asking yourself the questions, "Is this a STEMI? Why or why not?".

When reading the explanation, note the "Clinical Pearls" sections, which offer high-yield teaching points from each case. We have also included a cross-referenced index, which points you to common electrocardiographic patterns among the cases.

Introduction

BACKGROUND

The accurate diagnosis of an acute myocardial infarction (MI) in the first electrocardiogram (EKG) can guide decisions regarding urgent revascularization. Reducing the time to an accurate EKG diagnosis is essential. Survival and future morbidity after an acute MI depends upon how fast the occluded vessel can be opened. Various strategies have been proposed to reduce the time a vessel remains occluded. The Door-to-Balloon time is the single most important step and in reducing this time, an accurate and fast EKG diagnosis of an acute myocardial infarction is essential. The ability of the first responder, ER physician, Medical Student, Resident, Cardiology Fellow, and the attending to do so determines the outcome of the patient. Therefore it is imperative these providers are trained well to make the EKG diagnosis of an acute MI. Such an approach will provide the best outcome in these patients. For this purpose we developed an evidence-based EKG module to enhance the accuracy of EKG STEMI diagnosis.

The American College of Cardiology/American Heart Association/Heart Rhythm Society specify EKG criteria for ST elevation myocardial infarction (STEMI)[1] to identify candidates for emergent percutaneous coronary intervention (PCI). With much emphasis on reducing Door-to-Balloon time,[2,3] clinicians have only minutes to review the EKG at hand and make a diagnosis. An acceptable false positive rate in activating the cath lab of 5% has been proposed,[4,5]. This has been achieved in some centers[6] and is supported by a meta-analysis of serial EKG as a diagnostic tool.[7] Studies analyzing the field activations of cath labs by EMS providers show a false positive rate ranging up to 23%.[8] Confounding factors which contribute to this discrepancy include conditions which merit catheterization, but do not have the classic EKG findings associated with STEMI (STEMI-equivalents) and those which do no merit catheterization but whose EKG findings mimic STEMI (STEMI-mimics).

Electrocardiographic Characteristics

Classic STEMI

The current ACC/AHA guidelines specify the following criteria for diagnosing acute STEMI: ST-elevation (STE) in 2 anatomically contiguous leads >0.2mV (2mm) in leads V_1-V_3 and STE >0.1mV (1mm) in all other leads. At these thresholds, STE is the most effective ECG feature determining MI with a likelihood ratio of 13.1 (95% CI = 8.28–20.6)[9] and confer a sensitivity of 41.5% and specificity of 96.0%[1] for diagnosing STEMI. Electrocardiographic leads correlate with distinct anatomic regions of the heart, which, in turn, are perfused by specific coronary arteries. Changes in this perfusion pattern consequently result in ECG changes. This allows clinicians to reliably predict which arteries are occluded, helping guide intervention and prognostication.

Anterior STEMI
Anterior STEMI correlates to occlusion of the Left Anterior Descending (LAD) artery and is classically represented in the ECG by STE in leads V_1-V_4, with elevation ≥0.2mV (2mm) in V_2-V_3 specific for LAD STEMI.[1] ST elevation in V_1 to V_3 and in lead aVL in association with ST depression of more than 1mm in aVF indicates proximal occlusion of LAD.[10] New Right Bundle-Branch Block (RBBB) with a Q wave preceding the R wave in lead V_1 is a specific but insensitive marker of proximal occlusion of LAD in association with anterior septal MI.[10] ST elevation in leads V_2 to V_4 with elevation in the inferior leads suggest occlusion of the LAD distal to the origin of the first diagonal branch, in a vessel that wraps around the supply of the inferior apical region of the left ventricle.

Inferior STEMI
ST elevations in the inferior lead (leads II, III and aVF) is the main EKG finding. The right coronary artery (RCA) is the culprit vessel in 80% of the cases. A dominant left circumflex artery causes 20% of the inferior STEMIs. STE in lead III greater than lead II indicates RCA occlusion (sensitivity 88%, specificity 94%, positive predictive value 97%).[11,12] Proximal RCA occlusion can lead to right ventricular infarction, which is diagnosed by ST elevation of inferior leads and additional ST-elevation in lead V_1, the right-sided chest lead V_4R, or both.[1]

Lateral STEMI

ST elevations in the lateral leads (I, aVL, V5-V6) with reciprocal ST depression in the inferior leads is the typical EKG finding of lateral MIs. The diagonal branches of the LAD and the OM branches of the circumflex artery supply the lateral wall of the heart. Lateral STEMI due to circumflex artery occlusion can cause ST elevations in leads I, aVL, V_5 and V_6, but may also be seen in other leads (e.g. II and III). Some of the lateral STEMIs present without ST elevations.[13] There are three different patterns on the EKG of lateral infarctions: the infero-posterior-lateral pattern of the left circumflex occlusion described above, the anterior lateral pattern seen in a proximal LAD occlusion due to diagonal involvement (discussed in anterior STEMI segment) and the isolated lateral infarction due to a small branch supplying the lateral wall (OM, ramus intermedius or diagonal).

STEMI-Equivalents

New-Onset Left Bundle Branch Block (LBBB)

In acute settings, LBBB can be categorized as either a STEMI-mimic or a STEMI-equivalent. For decades, new onset LBBB was considered a STEMI-equivalent and the 1994 ACC/AHA and European guidelines strongly recommend reperfusion therapy.[14] Newer data reveal that most patients presenting with chest pain and LBBB are not having and acute MI. Therefore, treating all patients with LBBB and chest pain may expose patients to unnecessary procedures.[15]

Acute MI in Pre-existing LBBB

Normally, the QRS and ST segment in chronic LBBB are discordant. The Sgarbossa criteria describe QRS/ST concordance (with STE ≥1mm in ≥1 lead) to be the best predictor of acute infarction in known LBBB[16] (20% sensitivity and 98% specificity).[17] Extremely discordant ST deviation (>5 mm) is also suggestive of myocardial infarction in the presence of LBBB.

Posterior MI

Posterior MI is commonly seen in inferior STEMI. Isolated posterior MI presents with ST-depression ≥0.5mm in leads V_1-V_3. Associated T-waves are either upright or inverted and tall R-waves in V_1-V_2 may be present, although not always seen immediately. Because of the heterogeneous causes of ST-depression, the recommendation is to use additional posterior leads (V_7, V_9) to detect ST depression ≥0.5mm.[1,18]

Left Main Coronary Artery Occlusion (LMCO)
Acute LMCO is rapidly fatal. In a cath lab registry analysis of PCI cases from 2004-2008 LMCO represented .035% of all cases.[19] STE >0.5mm in aVR and, typically, greater than the STE in V_1, is 75% sensitive and 75% specific for LMCO.[20,21] Additionally, a 2009 AHA scientific statement[1] and a 2010 international consensus document[22] suggest similar criteria for acute LMCO: ST-depression in 6–8 leads, maximal in V_4-V_6, and associated ST-elevation in aVR and V_1, as above also suggest LMCO.

Wellen's Syndrome
Patients with a high grade proximal LAD stenosis, may develop the so-called Wellen's syndrome and are at very high risk of developing acute anterior infarction. Biphasic or inverted T waves in leads V_2-V_3 is diagnostic of this condition, indicating urgent PCI.[23]

Hyperacute T waves
One of the earliest ECG changes after the onset of an acute coronary artery occlusion are very tall, tented T-waves, or "Hyperacute T Waves".[24] These are rarely seen given their rapid disappearance or evolution to STE. However, when present, clinicians should strongly consider infarction in their differential and cath lab activation is recommended after ruling other causes of tall T-waves such as hyperkalemia.

STEMI-Mimics

ST-segment elevation can be a normal ECG finding, especially in young men.[25,26] The prevalence of STE in one or more of the precordial leads in normal ECGs in these studies is >90%. This underscores the importance of the clinical history and examination, which help to place the ECG in context.

LBBB
Making a diagnosis of myocardial infarction in LBBB is often difficult. The ST segment is often shifted in a discordant direction to the QRS in LBBB. A newly recognized LBBB with a clinical history consistent with myocardial infarction may be an indication for PCI[14]. The Sgarbossa criteria are specific for acute MI in

known LBBB: Concordant ST elevations > 1mm in leads with a positive QRS complex, concordant ST depressions > 1mm in V1-V3 or excessively discordant ST elevations > 5mm in leads with a negative QRS complex are part of the criteria.[16] Recognition of these differences is key to an accurate diagnosis.

Acute Pericarditis

Acute pericarditis manifests on the ECG as diffuse concave ST segment elevations throughout most leads with associated PR depression. Lead aVR may show reciprocal PR segment elevation and ST depression. Sinus tachycardia is commonly present due to pain. This contrasts STEMI where anatomically correlated leads will show convex ST segment elevations, often with reciprocal ST-depression elsewhere.[27,28]

Hyperkalemia

Electrocardiographic changes secondary to hyperkalemia are well known. The earliest sings are peaked T-waves. As the potassium continues to rise, small P-waves, conduction abnormalities (high grade AV block, junctional or ventricular escape rhythms) and very wide and bizarre QRS complex with impressive ST segment abnormalities are reported.[29]

Brugada Syndrome

Brugada syndrome is a genetic disorder linked to cardiac sodium-channel gene mutation. It occurs in patients with structurally normal hearts and is associated with a high incidence of sudden cardiac death.[30,31] The typical Coved ST segment elevation of greater than 2 mm in leads V_1-V2 followed by an inverted T wave can be easily confused with an ST elevation MI. Another pattern noted in Brugada patients is a saddleback ST segment shape.

Left Ventricular Hypertrophy

There are many EKG criteria for diagnosing LVH. The most commonly used are the Sokolov-Lyon criteria with deep S waves in V1 and tall R waves in V5 or V6 > 35 mm.[32] Cornell criteria S-wave in V3 + R-wave in avL > 28 mm in men and > 20 mm in women has a 98% specificity.[33] The thickened LV wall leads to prolonged depolarization and delayed repolarization with marked ST and T wave abnormalities that are frequently mistaken for acute infarction patterns. The ST segment tends to be concave in shape in LVH patients, compared to a convex ST-segment seen in STEMI patients.

Early Repolarization

Early repolarization has been a recognized normal variant since 1936.[34] Concave ST elevations in the mid-precordial leads V_2-V_5, most prominent in leads V_3-V_4, and notching of the J-point is present, which is atypical for acute infarction.

Pulmonary Embolism (PE)

The most common ECG finding in PE is sinus tachycardia. ST elevations have been reported in many patients with PE. S1 QIII TIII is a classic finding for PE but found in only 20% of patients. Right heart strain with T wave inversions along the right precordial leads (V1-V4) and inferior leads can be seen and reported as the most specific finding in PE. Incomplete or complete RBBB, dominant R wave in V1 and right axis deviation can occur. In massive pulmonary embolism, a pseudo-infarction pattern may manifest on the ECG due to right ventricular pressure overload and/or dilation.[35,36]

Takotsubo

Also known as Broken Heart Syndrome, is typically seen in post-menopausal woman with severe emotional distress. The amount of ST segment elevation on leads V4-V6 is usually greater than the ones on V1-V3. There are no reciprocal ST segment changes and no Q waves present on the presenting EKGs. Coronary angiography is usually performed to distinguish STEMI from Takotusbo cardiomyopathy. [37]

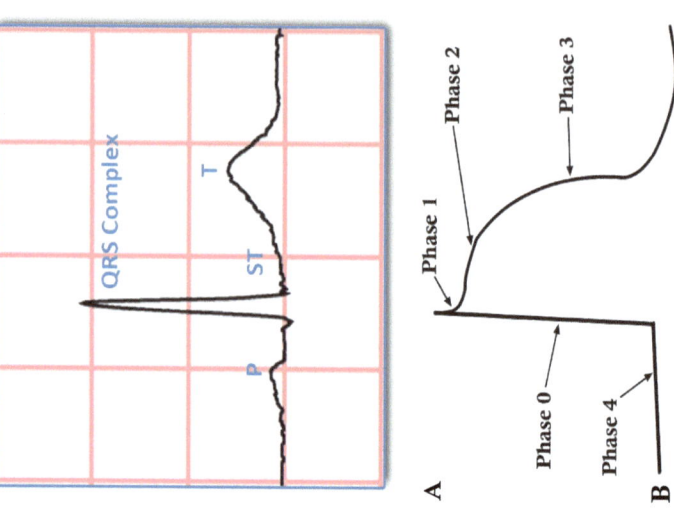

Fig. 2 A, Timing of normal EKG action potential. **B,** The cardiac myocyte depolarization-repolarization phases. Phase 0 is the rapid depolarization phase, followed by phase 1 (rapid repolarization) and then 2, the 'plateau' phase. Phase 3 is the repolarization phase that restores the membrane potential to its resting value. Phase 4 is the resting potential.

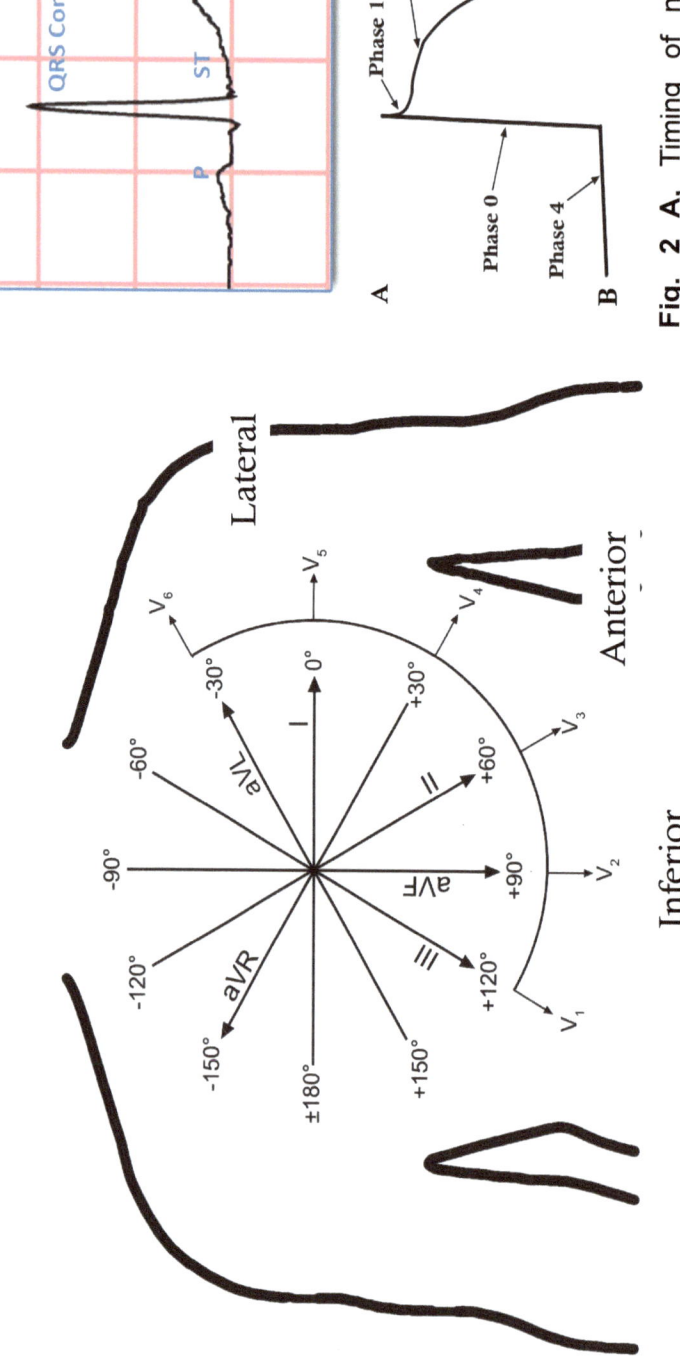

Fig. 1 The 12-lead EKG and its vectors.

Anterior leads = V2-V4
Lateral leads = I, aVL, V5-V6
Inferior leads = II, III and aVF
Right ventricular leads = aVR and V1

ABBREVIATIONS

A/W	Associated with	LV	Left Ventricle
AMI	Acute Myocardial Infarction	LVH	Left Ventricular Hypertrophy
AV	Atrioventricular	MI	Myocardial Infarction
C/O	Complains of	NICM	Non-Ischemic Cardiomyopathy
C/W	Consistent with	NSAIDs	Non-Steroidal Anti-inflammatory Drugs
CAD	Coronary Artery Disease	OM	Obtuse Marginal Coronary Artery
CHF	Congestive Heart Failure	PVC	Premature Ventricular Complex
CKD	Chronic Kidney Disease	PPV	Positive Predictive Value
COPD	Chronic Obstructive Pulmonary Disease	RA	Right Atrium
DM	Diabetes Mellitus	RBBB	Right Bundle Branch Block
EF	Ejection Fraction	RCA	Right Coronary Coronary Artery
EKG	Electrocardiogram	RV	Right Ventricle
ER	Emergency Room	S/P	Status Post
GERD	Gastroesophageal Reflux Disease	STD	ST Segment Depression
H/O	History of	STE	ST Segment Elevation
HIV	Human Immunodeficiency Virus	STEMI	ST Segment Elevation Myocardial Infarction
HLD	Hyperlipidemia	SVG	Saphenous Vein Graft
HTN	Hypertension	TC	Takotsubo Cardiomyopathy
IVDA	Intravenous Drug Abuse	TWI	T-Wave Inversion
LA	Left Atrium	VF	Ventricular Fibrillation
LAD	Left Anterior Descending Coronary Artery	VT	Ventricular Tachycardia
LBBB	Left Bundle Branch Block	Y.O.	Year-Old
LCx	Left Circumflex Coronary Artery		
LIMA	Left Internal Mammary Artery		

Normal Coronary Angiogram

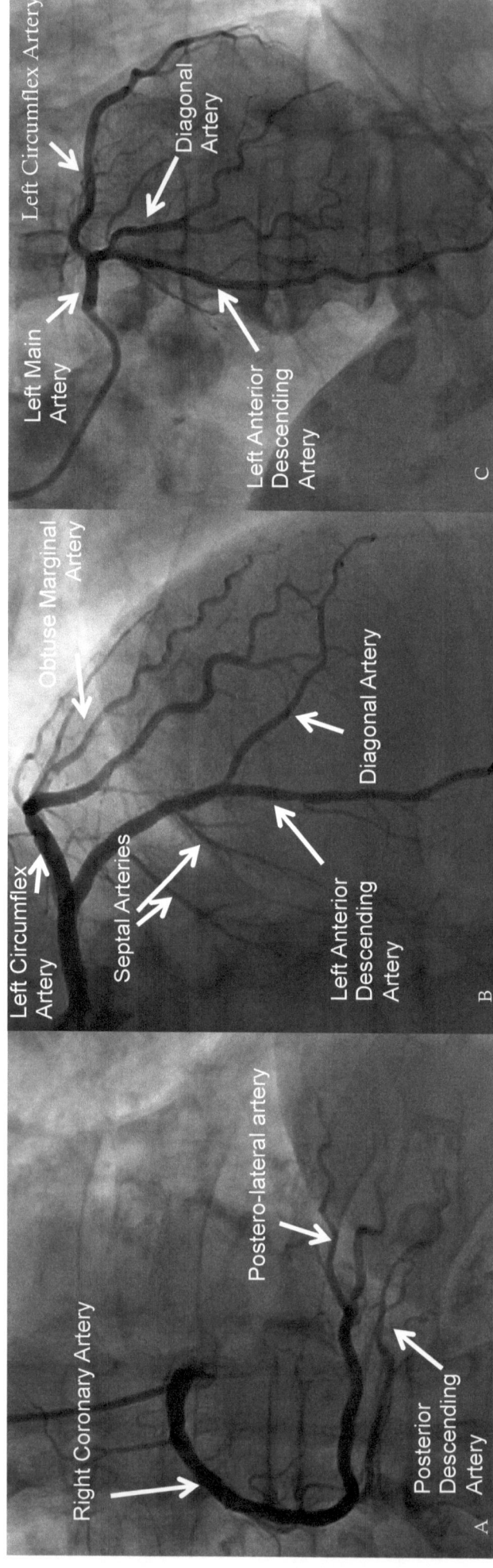

Fig. 3 Cardiac catheterization images displaying normal coronary anatomy. **A**: Left-Anterior Oblique view of the RCA, **B**: AP Cranial view of the LAD and LCx, **C**: Left-Anterior Oblique Cranial view of the LAD and LCx.

12

Normal EKG

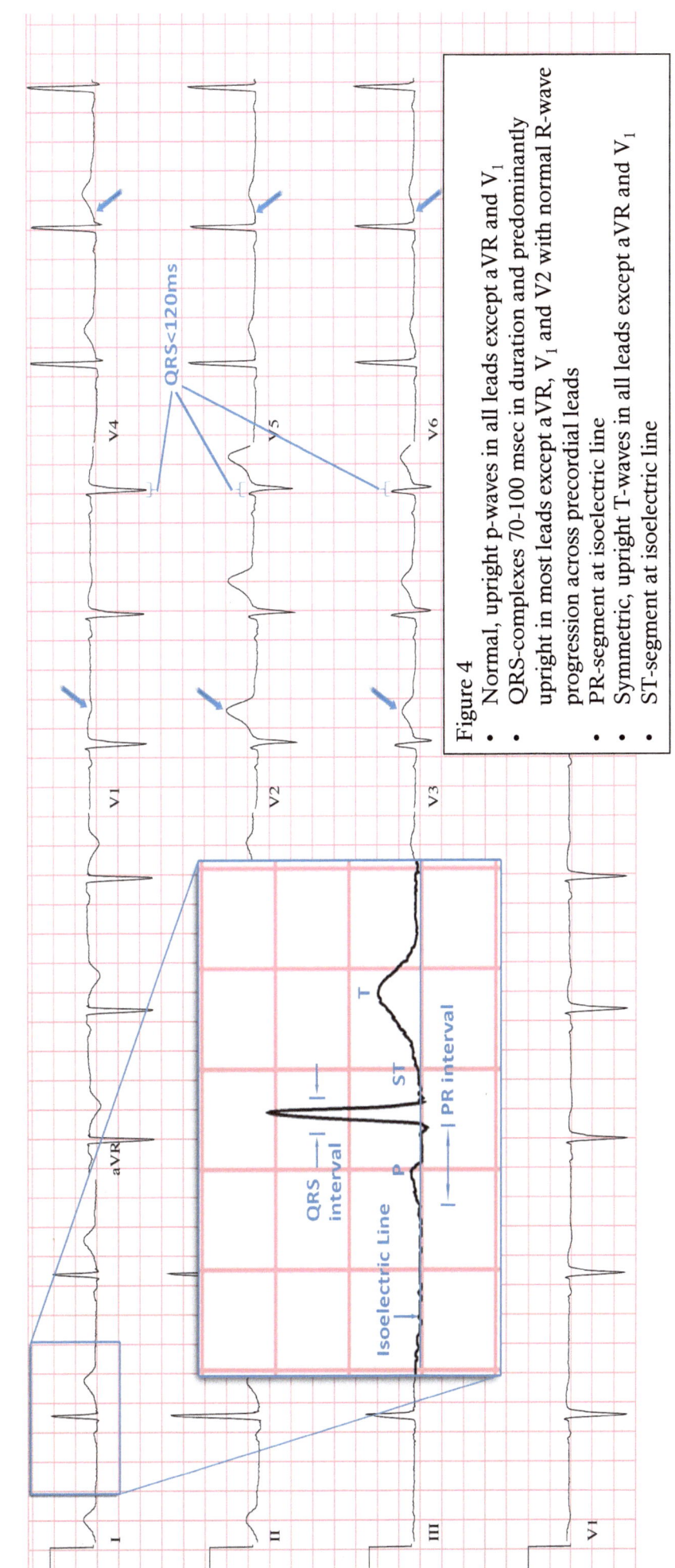

Figure 4
- Normal, upright p-waves in all leads except aVR and V_1
- QRS-complexes 70-100 msec in duration and predominantly upright in most leads except aVR, V_1 and V2 with normal R-wave progression across precordial leads
- PR-segment at isoelectric line
- Symmetric, upright T-waves in all leads except aVR and V_1
- ST-segment at isoelectric line

CLASSIC STEMIS

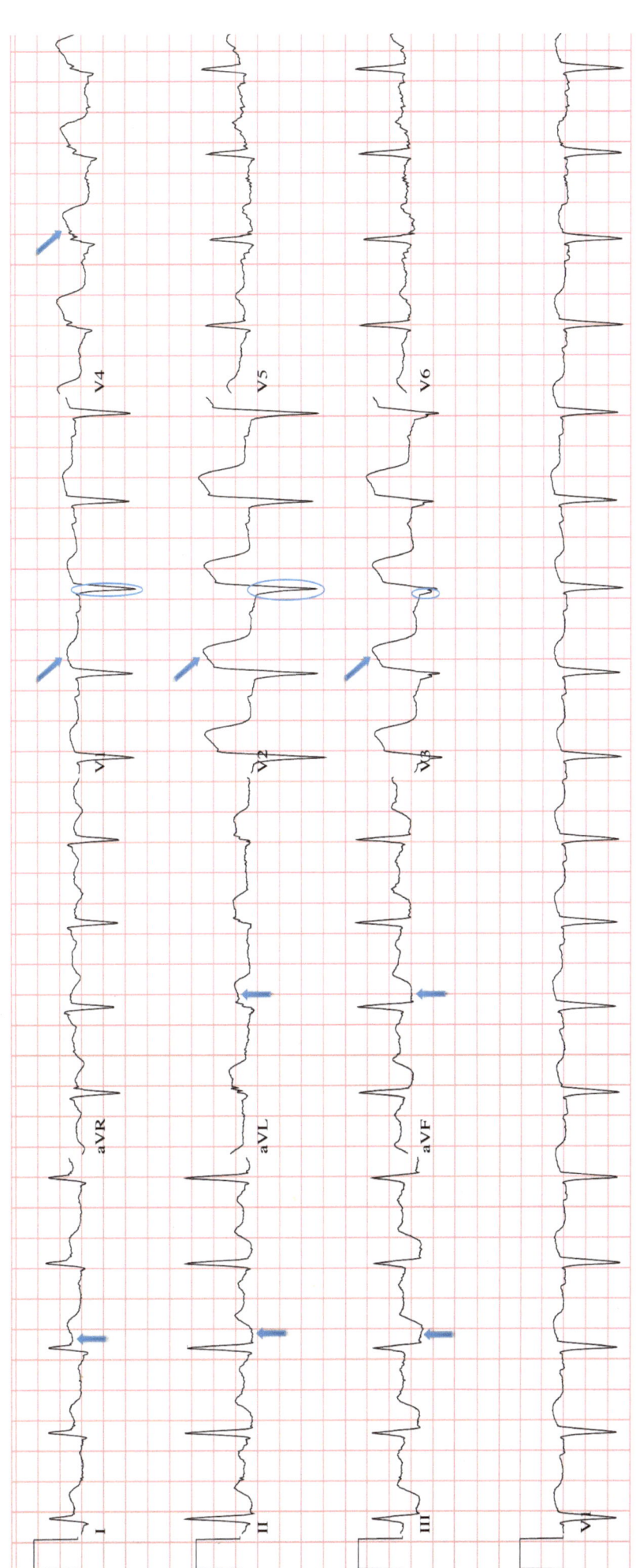

15

Case 1: A 48 y.o. man with tobacco use c/o intermittent chest pain and diaphoresis for one hour

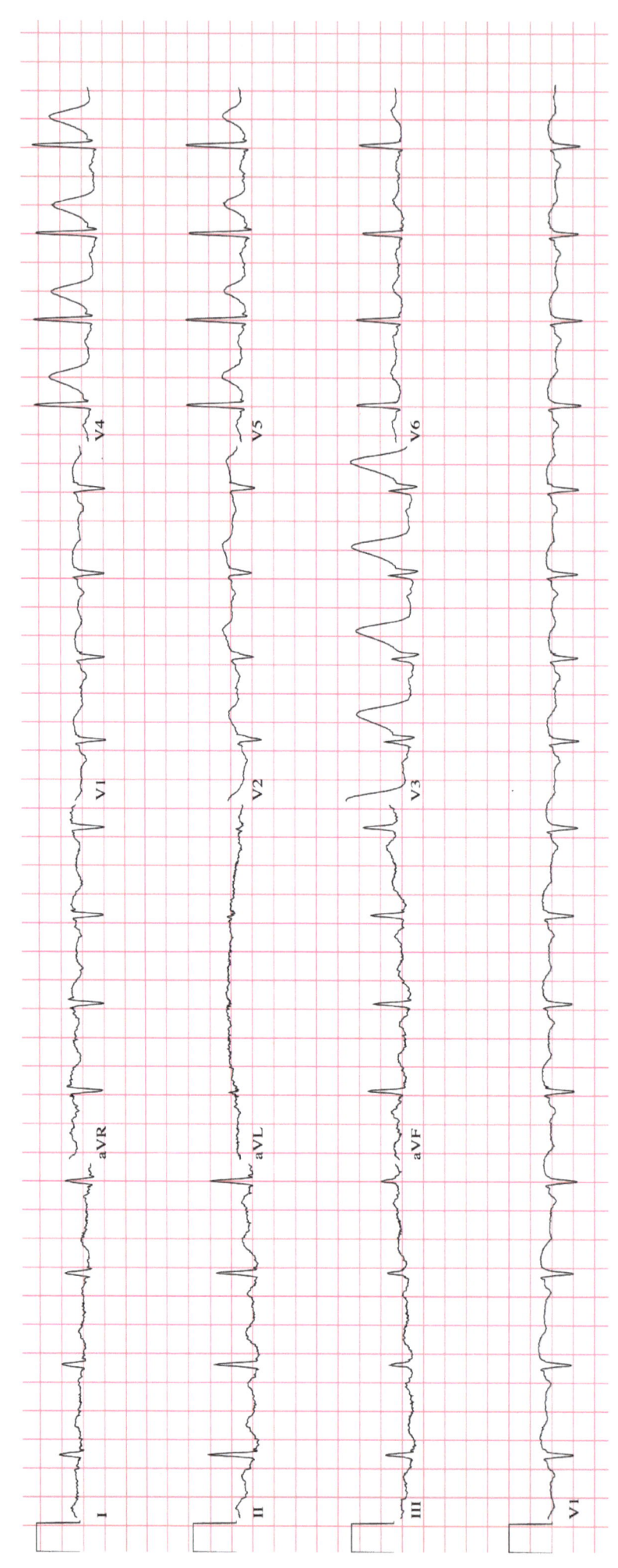

Anterior-Septal Myocardial Injury

Features:

- New ST segment elevation at the J point of V1-V4 consistent with Anterior Myocardial Injury

- Anterior pattern- STE in V_2-V_4 is specific for LAD occlusion. [1,10,38]

- Septal involvement- STE in V_1 indicates occlusion of the septal perforators[10,39]

Other findings in this case:

- Q waves are absent
- Q waves appear after the second hour of chest pain[40]

Clinical Pearl:

- Myocardial Injury = ST segment elevation and absent Q waves

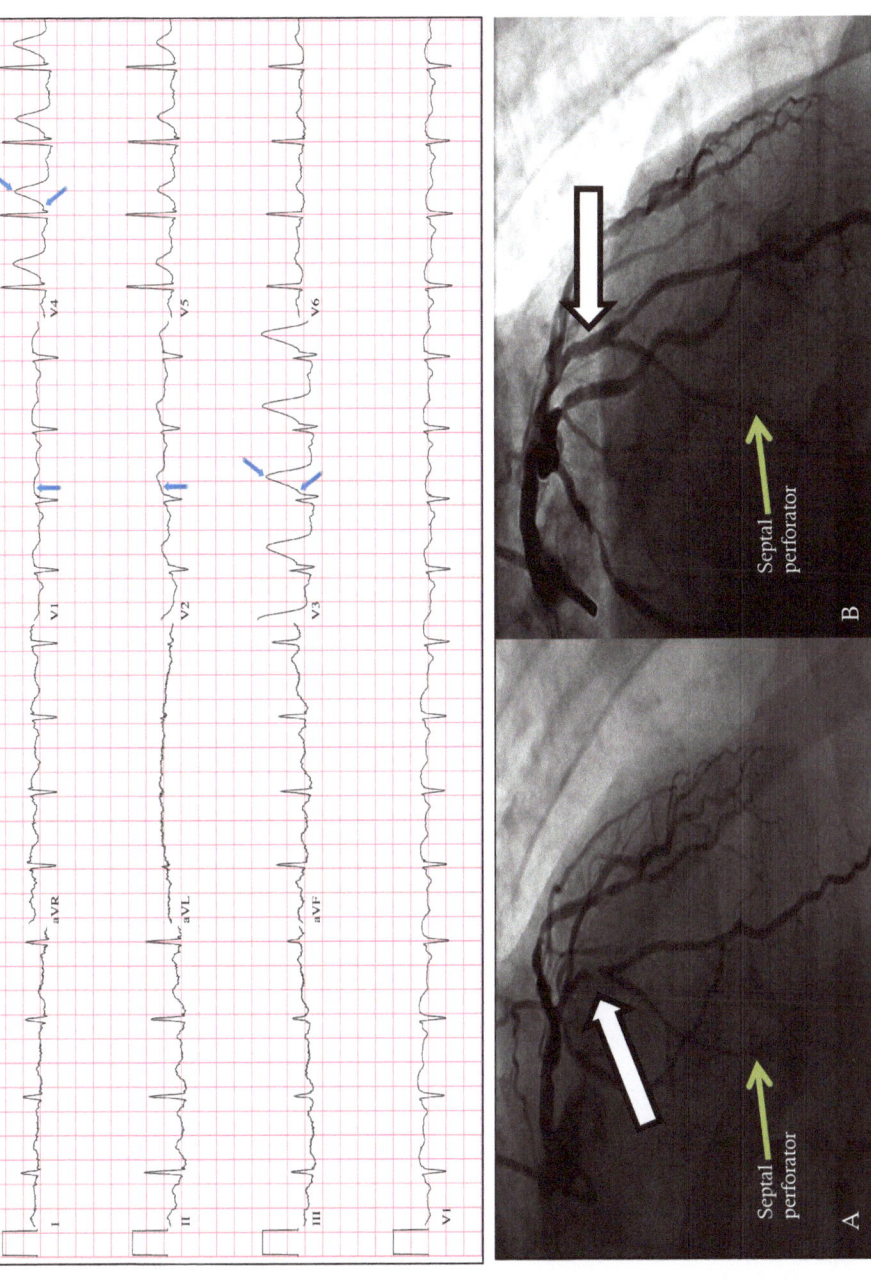

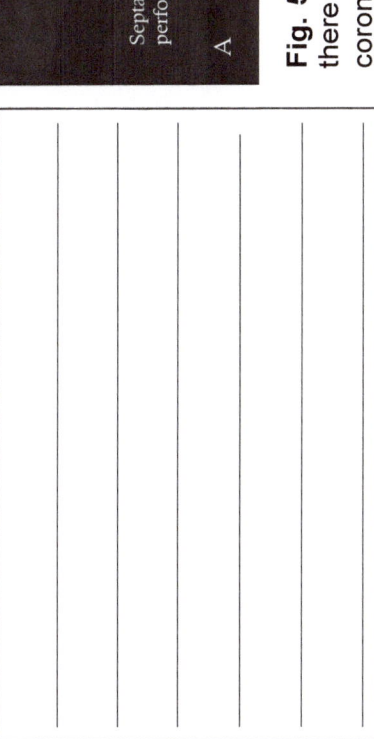

Fig. 5 A, Pre-intervention cath image showing a 95% Mid-LAD occlusion (large arrow). Note there is still some blood flow distal to the stenosis. **B,** Post-intervention showing restored coronary blood flow (large arrow). Note the second septal perforator branch (small arrow).

17

Case 2: A 47 y.o. man with HTN c/o chest pressure for 2 hours

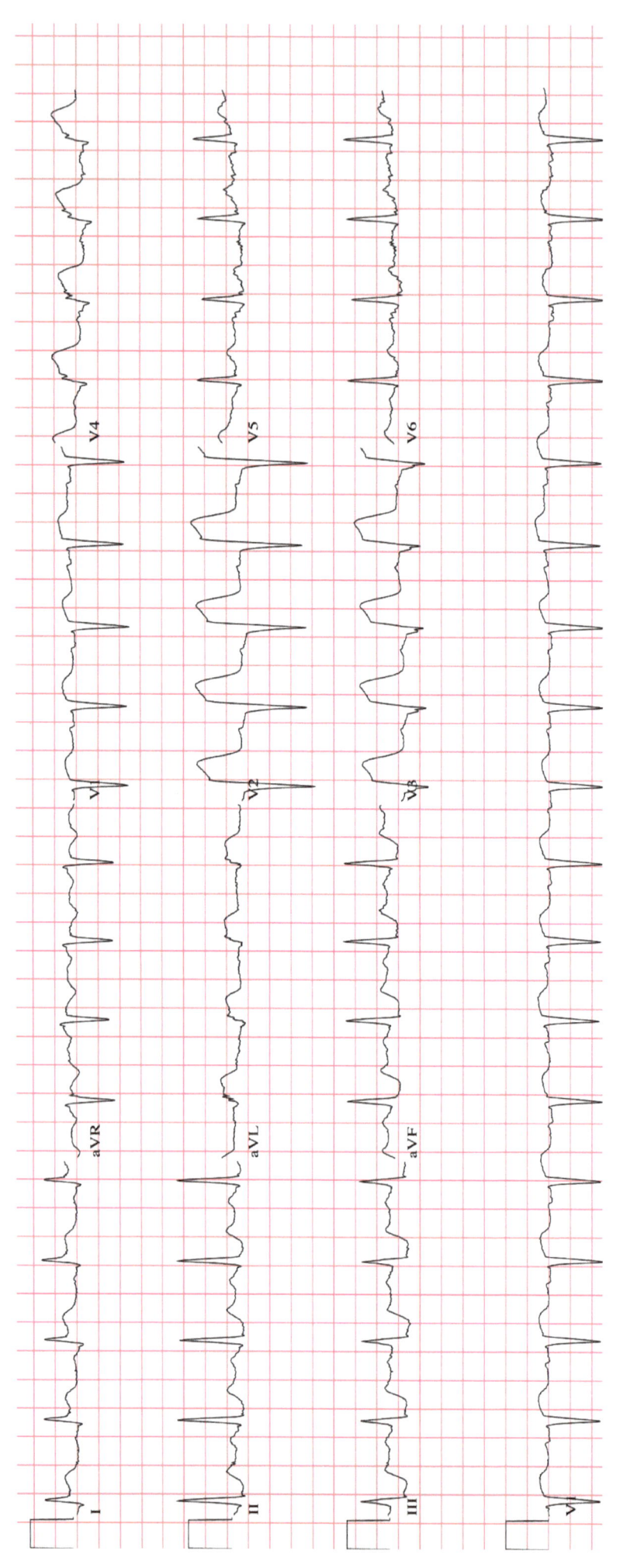

Antero-Septal STEMI
LAD occlusion proximal to diagonal

Features:

- Anterior pattern- STE in V_2–V_4 ≥ 2 mm is specific for LAD occlusion[10,38,41]

- STE in V_1 indicates occlusion of septal perforators and c/w septal involvement [10,39]

- Proximal LAD occlusion- Anterior pattern and STE in V_1 combined with reciprocal STD > 1mm in inferior leads (II, III, aVF) [38,41]

- Lateral STE in I, aVL indicates occlusion proximal to the diagonal branches of the LAD, which supply the lateral wall of the left ventricle[10,42]

Clinical Pearls:

- To code for an anteroseptal MI, abnormal Q waves must be present in leads V1, V2 _and_ V3.

- Q-waves in V_1-V_4 indicate longer than 2 hour duration of ischemia [40]

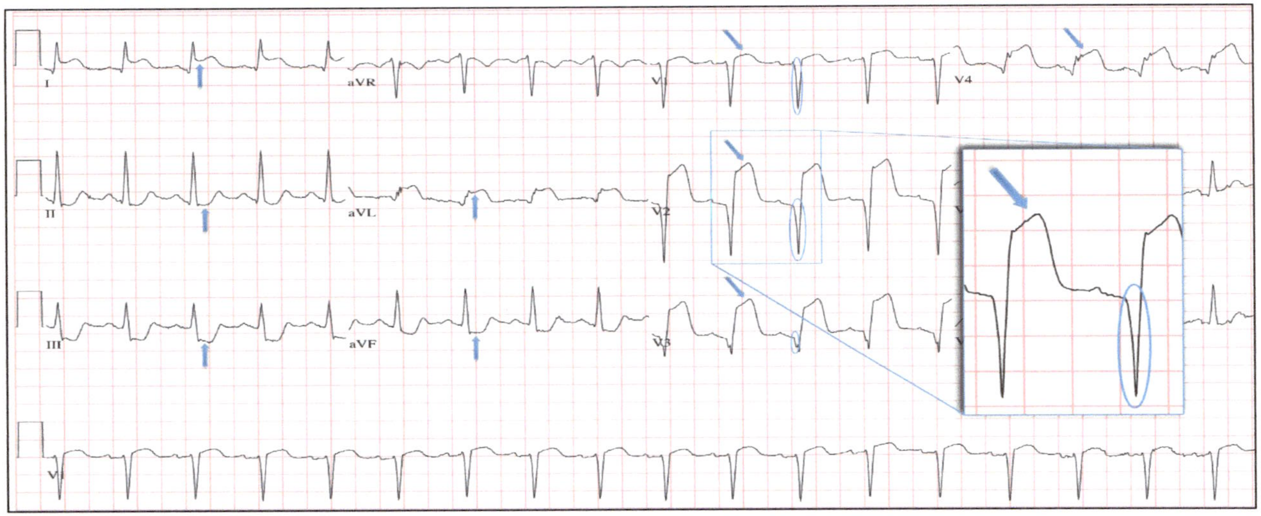

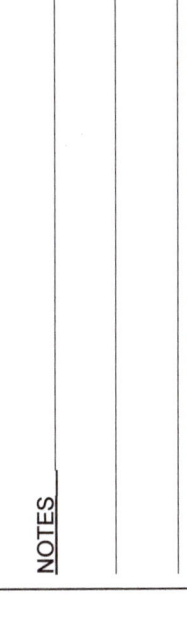

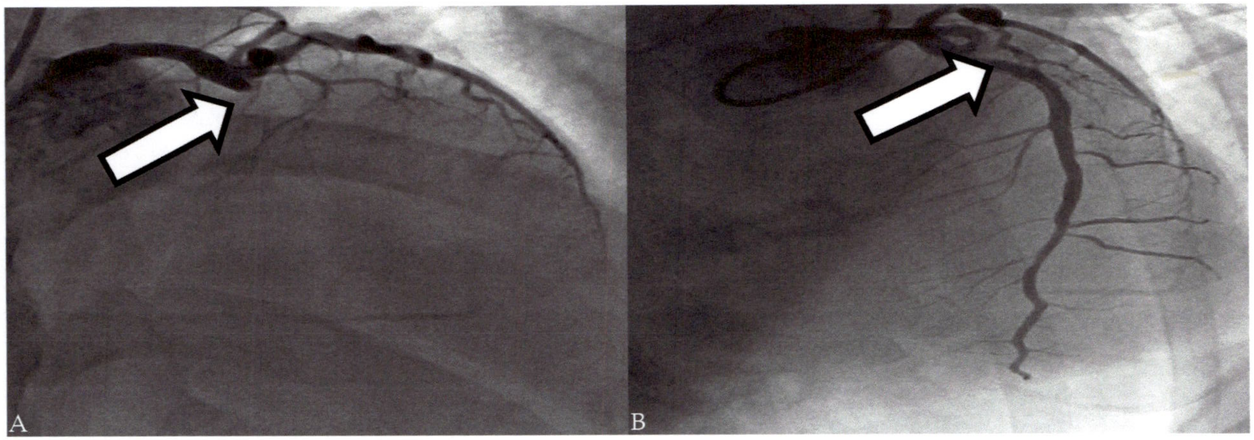

Fig. 6 A, Pre-intervention catheterization image showing a 100% Proximal-LAD occlusion (large arrow). **B,** Post-intervention showing restored coronary blood flow (large arrow).

NOTES

Case 3: A 51 y.o. man with HTN c/o 2 days of chest pain radiating to his neck and jaw, troponin of 40

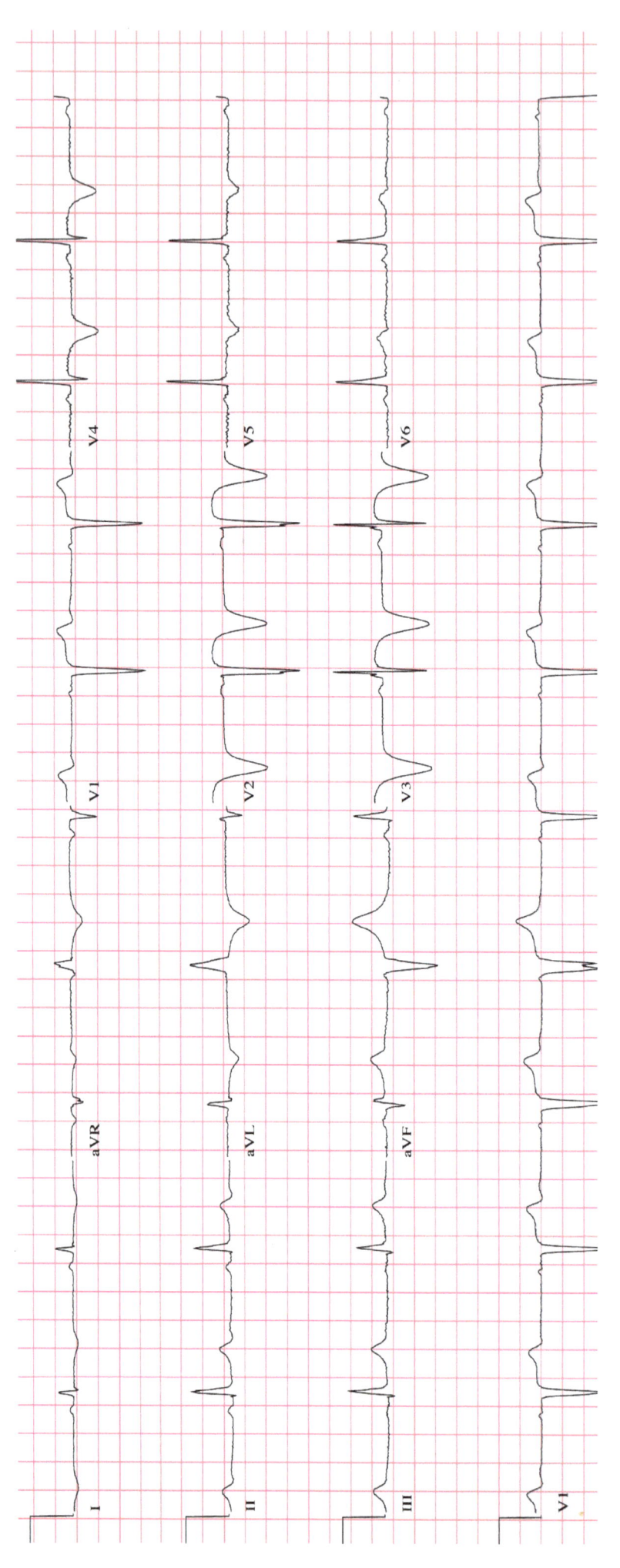

Anterior MI (age recent)

Features:

- Anterior pattern- STE in V_2–V_4 ≥ 2 mm is specific for LAD occlusion[10,38,41]
  - STE in V_2–V_3 suffices to locate this to the anterior myocardium
  - Note the convex upwards, or "tombstoning" shape of the STE
- Ischemic TWI pattern- Deep, symmetric TWI in V_2–V_5 supports an ischemic cause

Other findings in this case:

- Presence of R-wave and absence of Q-wave in V_3 indicates injury rather than transmural infarct
- TWI in I, aVL indicates some lateral involvement
- Injured myocardium is more likely to have ectopic depolarization, notice PVC as the 4th beat.

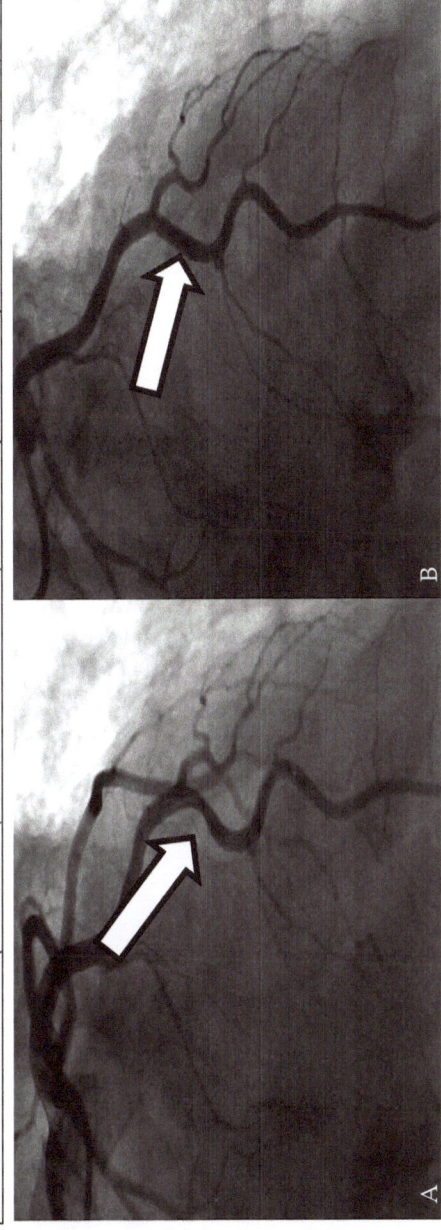

Fig. 7 A, Pre-intervention cath image showing a 50-60% Mid-LAD stenosis with thrombus (large arrow). **B**, Post-intervention showing restored coronary blood flow (large arrow).

NOTES

Case 4: A 37 y.o. woman with HTN c/o chest pain while exercising

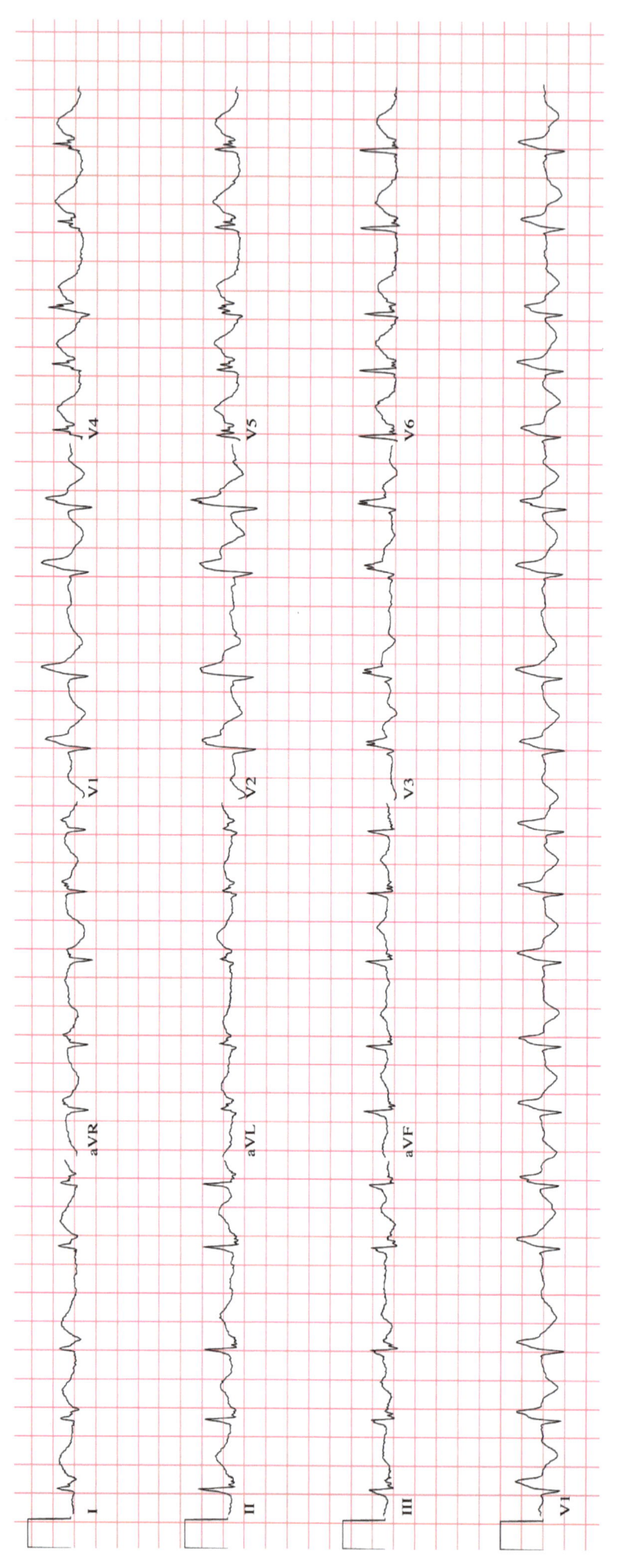

Antero-Lateral STEMI with RBBB

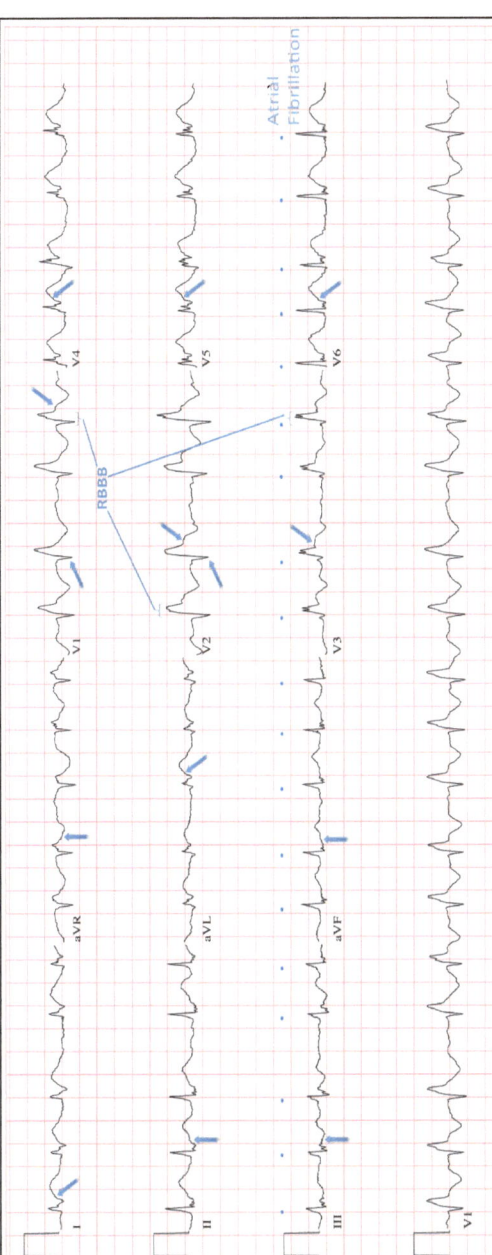

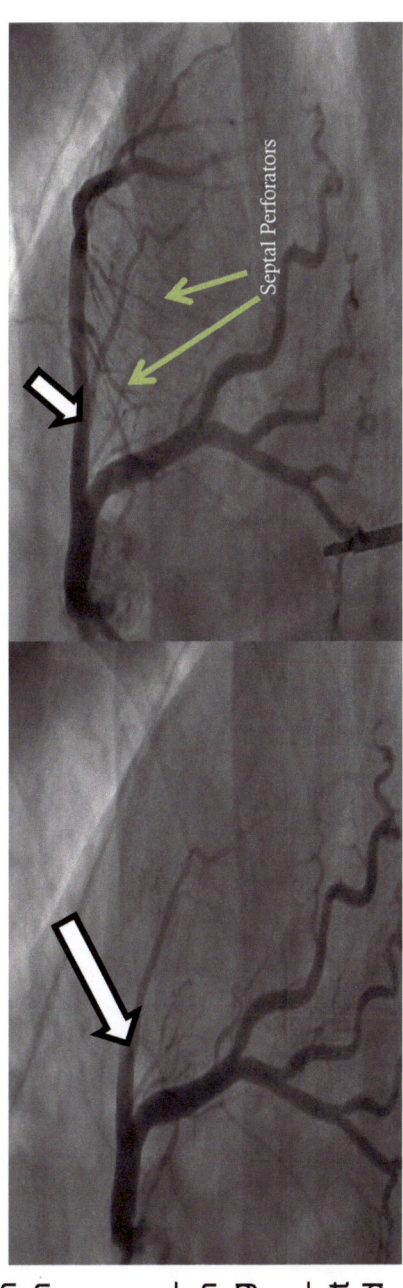

Features:

- New RBBB with Q wave in V1 is specific for occlusion proximal to the septal perforators.[39]
- RBBB is associated with negative ST and T waves in V1, because of ST elevations there is pseudonormalization of the ST segment.
- Anterior pattern- STE in V_2-V_4 ≥ 2 mm is specific for LAD occlusion[1,10,38,41]
- STE throughout the precordial leads V_2-V_6 indicates an extensive MI [43]
- Lateral pattern- STE in I, aVL, V_5, V_6 indicate lateral wall involvement[13,41]
- Septal pattern- STE in V_1, aVR and STD in inferior leads II, III, aVF indicate occlusion proximal to first septal perforator[1,10]

Clinical Pearls:

- Atrial fibrillation can occur due to volume-pressure overload of the LA caused by an acutely dilated hypo-functioning LV or during periods of adrenergic stress.
- Risk of progression to 3rd degree AV block- 30% if only RBBB present, 45% if RBBB + left anterior hemiblock present, 60% if RBBB and left posterior hemiblock present.[44]

Fig. 8 A, Pre-intervention cath image showing a 100% Proximal-LAD occlusion (large arrow). **B,** Post-intervention showing restored coronary blood flow (large arrow) with now-perfused septal perforators (thin arrows)

Case 5: A 49 y.o man with HTN, DM, and HLD c/o of intermittent chest pain that has become persistent

Antero-Apical STEMI

Features:

- Antero-apical pattern- STE in V_3–V_6 and STE in II, III, aVF [10,45]
- Wrap-around LAD- STE in both V_2-V_4 (anterior) and II, III, aVF (inferior leads) indicate a distal occlusion of an LAD that perfuses the infero-apical wall [45,46] (Fig. 11B)

Other findings in this case:

- Pseudonormalization in V_1 and V_2 due to RBBB
  - The RBBB leads to a falsely normalized ST-segment, which without it would appear as STE. (See case 5)
  - RBBB is pre-existing because the occlusion is distal to the first septal perforator (Fig. 11A)
  - Q-waves noted in III and aVF indicate longer duration of ischemia

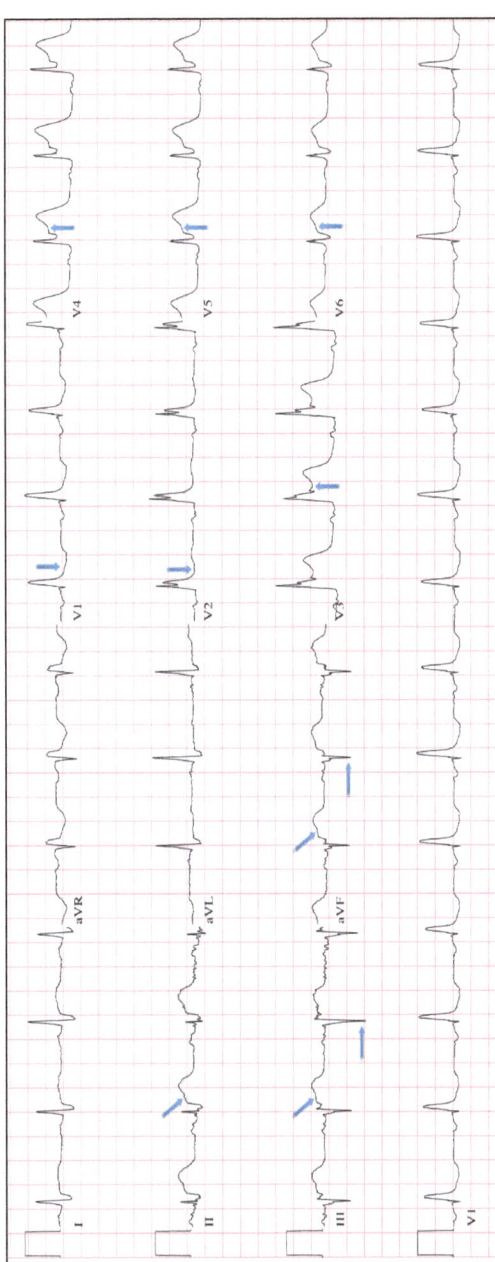

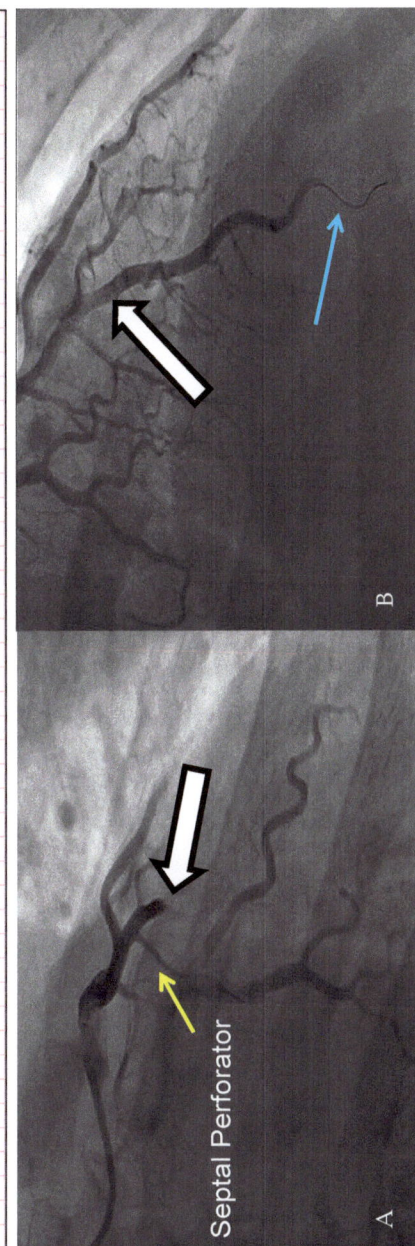

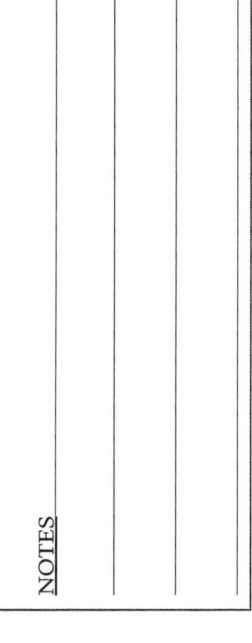

Septal Perforator

A   B

Fig. 9 A, Pre-intervention catheterization image showing a 100% Mid-LAD occlusion (large arrow). **B**, Post-intervention showing restored blood flow (large arrow). Catheter is seen in wrap-around LAD (small arrow)

<u>NOTES</u>

25

Case 6: A 52 y.o. man c/o 30 minutes of chest pain and diaphoresis s/p VF arrest

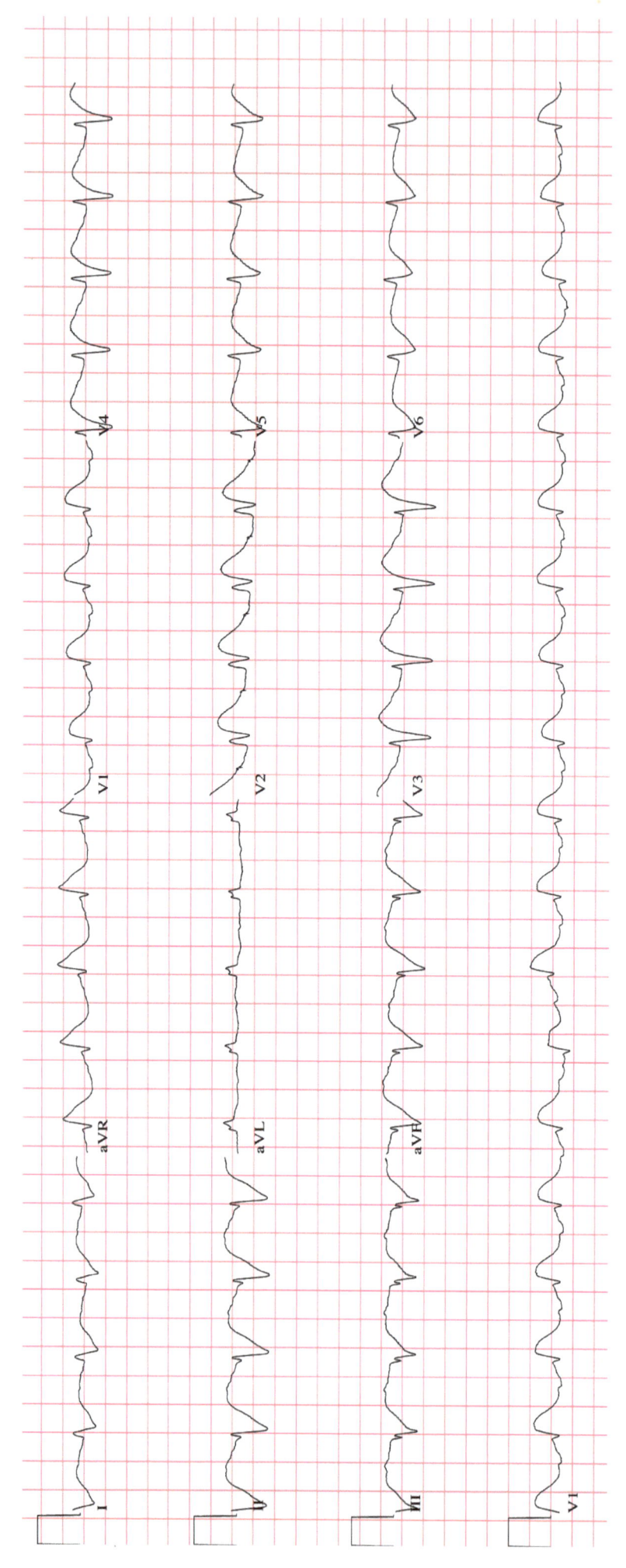

Left Main Equivalent

Features:
- Left main or left main equivalent- STE in aVR ≥ 1 mm and STE in aVR ≥ V$_1$ (81% sensitivity, 80% specificity) [20,47]

Other findings in this case:
- Anterior pattern- STE in V$_1$-V$_4$ [1,10,38,41]
- Septal pattern- STE in V$_1$, aVR [10,39,48]
- Injury pattern- Lack of Q waves in anterior leads indicates more recent onset.
- Reciprocal STD in I, aVL, V$_5$, V$_6$
- Sinus tachycardia- note P-waves in V$_1$

Clinical Pearls:
- Indicators of a large infarction:
- Terminal QRS distortion with STE in AMI indicates larger infarct size with more rapid progression to myocardial necrosis. QRS appears to mimic a RBBB, the large degree of STE makes it appear wide [49]
- Increased magnitude of and number of leads with STE correlate to the amount of myocardium at risk and the prognostic outcome [43,50]

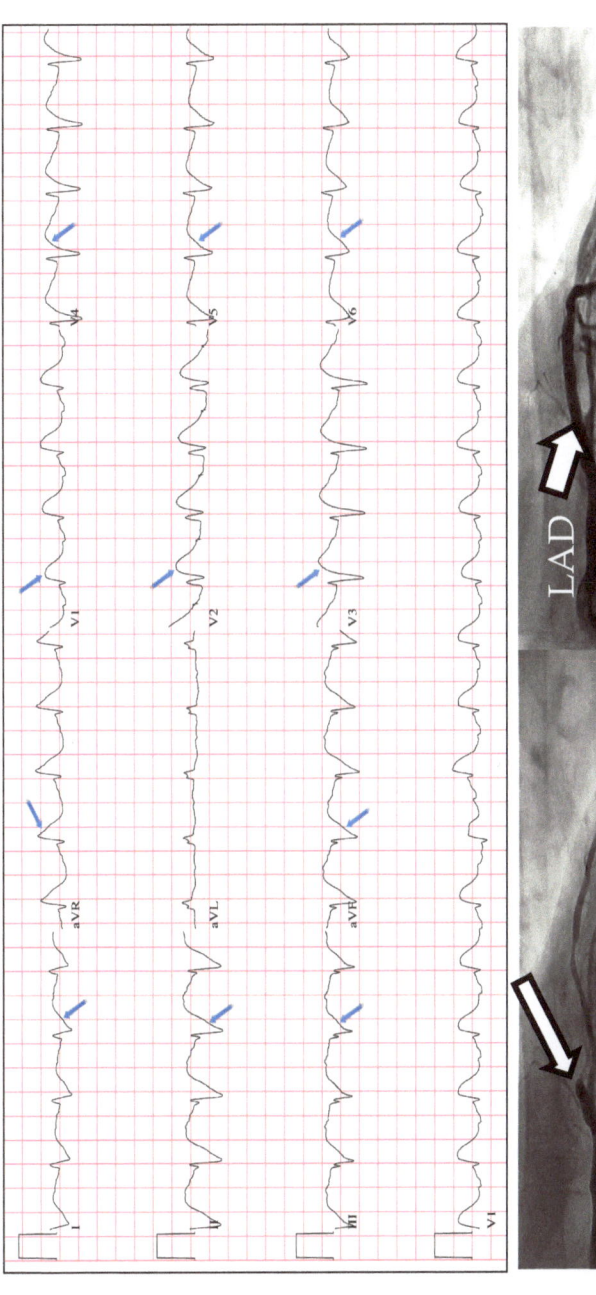

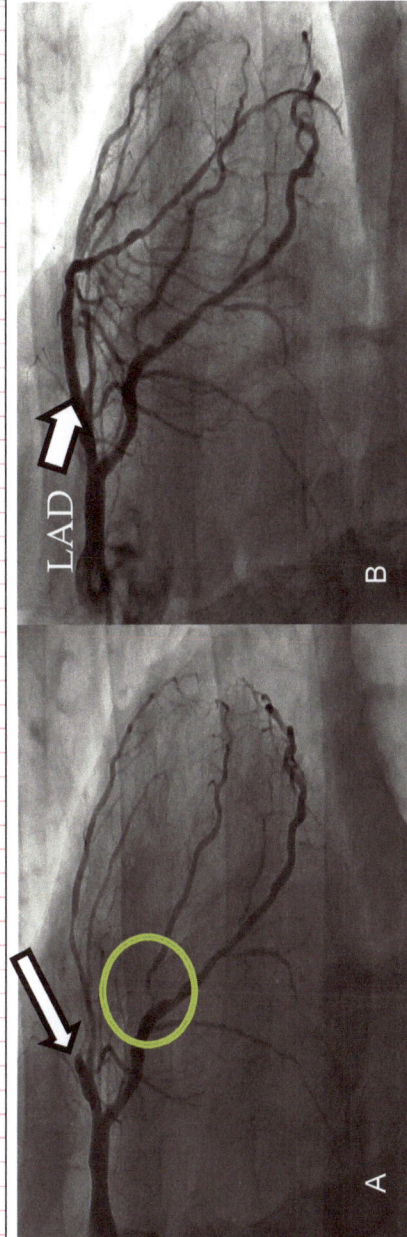

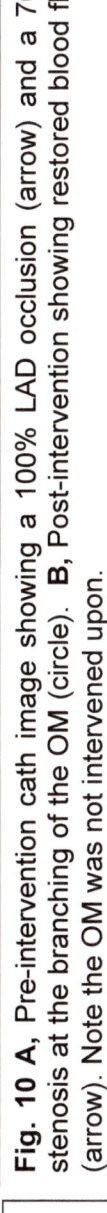

Fig. 10 A, Pre-intervention cath image showing a 100% LAD occlusion (arrow) and a 70% stenosis at the branching of the OM (circle). **B,** Post-intervention showing restored blood flow (arrow). Note the OM was not intervened upon.

NOTES

Case 7: A 62 y.o. man c/o chest pain while on a treadmill at the gym

Infero-Lateral STEMI with Fixed-Coupling PVCs

Features:

- Inferior pattern- STE in II, III, aVF is the classic EKG manifestation of an inferior MI[12,48]

- Lateral pattern- STE in leads I indicates some lateral involvement[13,44,48]

Other findings in this case:

- Fixed coupled PVCs are triggered by ischemia [48,51,52]

Clinical Pearl:

- LCx infarct can cause an inferior infarct. Comparing the STE in II and III suggests whether the culprit artery is the RCA or in the LCx territory. STE in lead III not > lead II and lateral STE points to an occlusion in the LCx system [53]

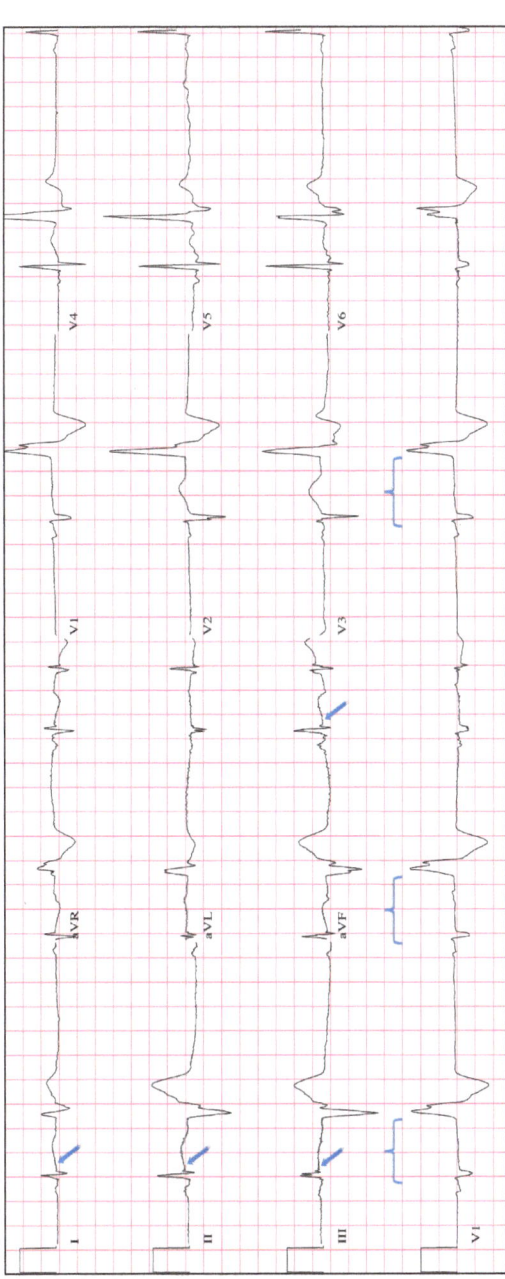

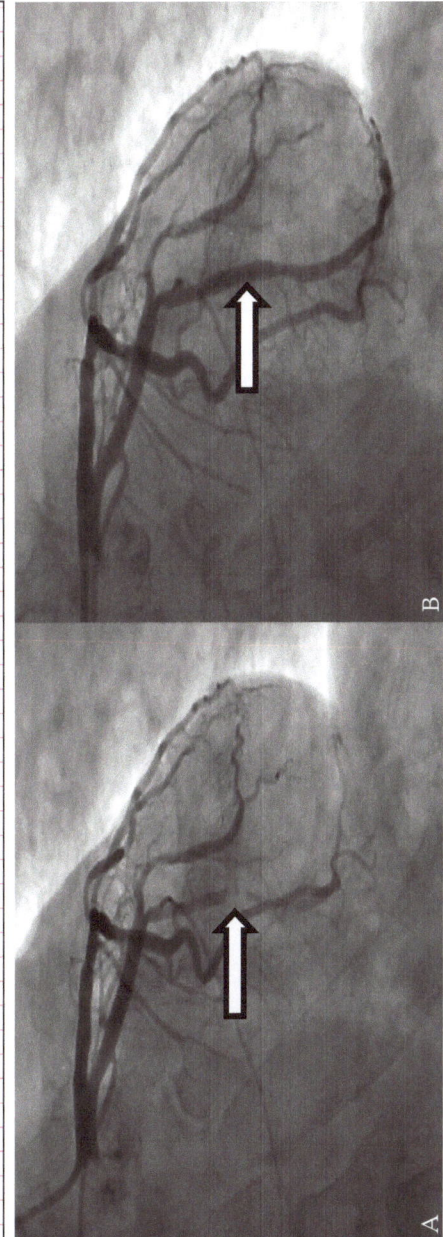

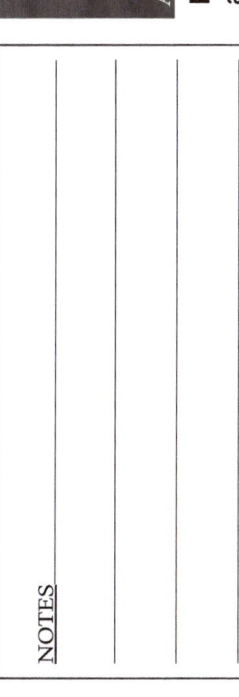

Fig. 11 A, Pre-intervention catheterization image showing a 100% OM1 occlusion (large arrow). **B,** Post-intervention showing restored blood flow (large arrow).

NOTES

Case 8: A 60 y.o. man with HLD and GERD c/o chest pain that began while exercising

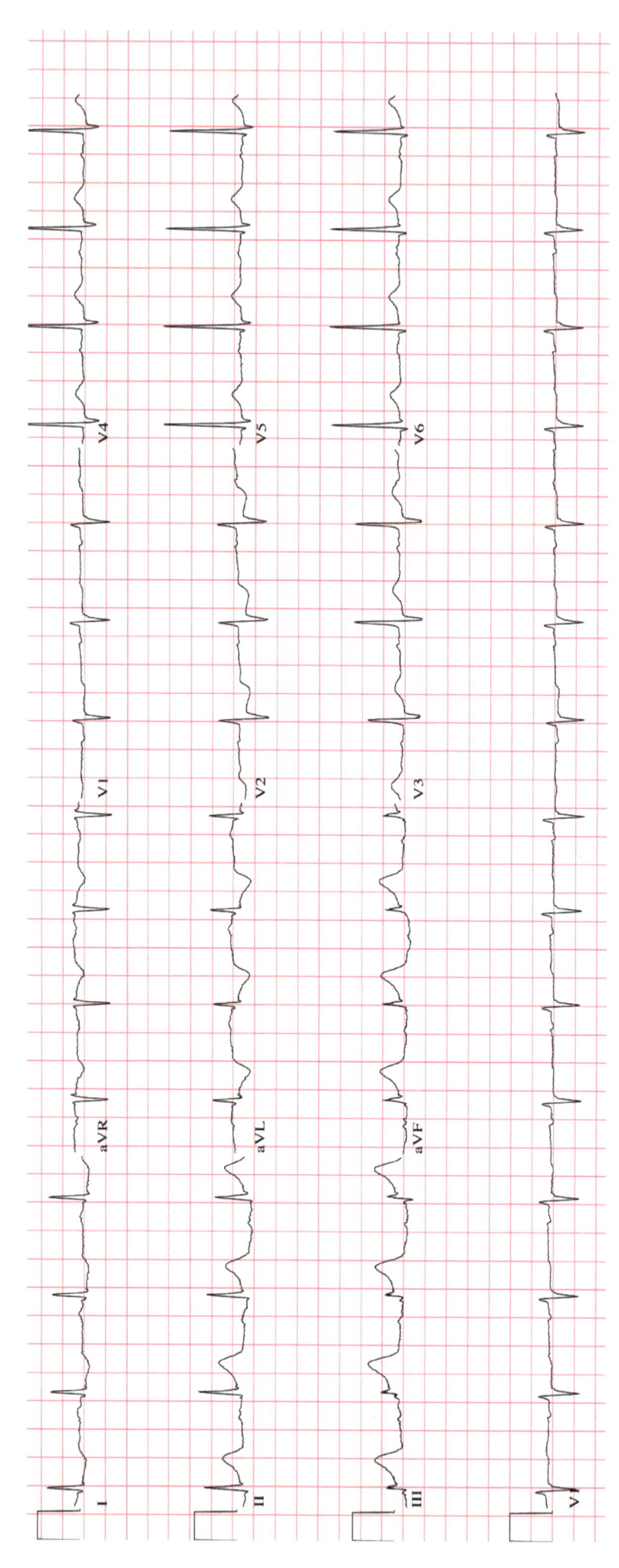

Infero-Posterior STEMI

Features:

- Inferior MI pattern- STE in II, III, aVF [12,48]
- Posterior MI – ST segment depression in V_1-V_2 in the setting of an inferior MI [1,54,55]
- Posterior infarct in inferior MI usually indicates a dominant RCA[1,44,48,56]
- Tall R-waves in V_1-V_3 are equivalent to Q-waves in the posterior wall, indicating longer time of ischemia [48,57]
- Reciprocal ST depressions in I and aVL indicates lateral involvement, which further supports a very dominant RCA [48]

Clinical Pearls:

- Comparing STE in II to III in inferior MIs can suggest whether the culprit artery is RCA or LCx. In this case, STE in III > II and STD > 1 mm in I and/or aVL has a sensitivity of 90% and a specificity of 71% for an RCA occlusion[1,11,12,38,44]
- It is important to code the ST segment depression present in leads V1 and V2 due to posterior MI.

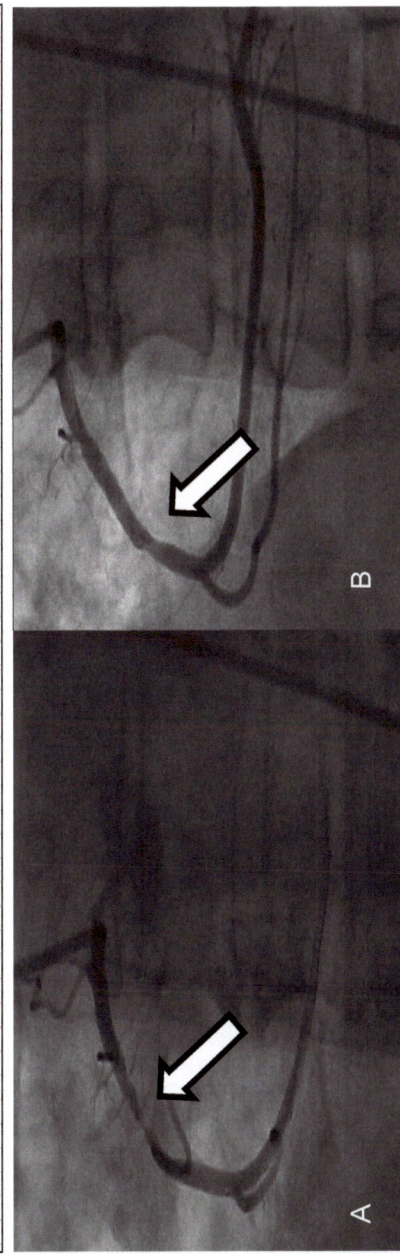

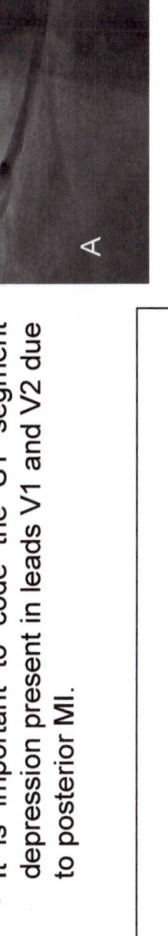

Fig. 12 A, Pre-intervention cath image showing RCA stenosis with thrombus (arrow). **B,** Post-intervention showing restored blood flow (arrow). Note this is a large caliber, dominant RCA.

NOTES

Case 9: A 49 y.o. woman with HTN c/o chest pain and then becomes hypotensive and bradycardic

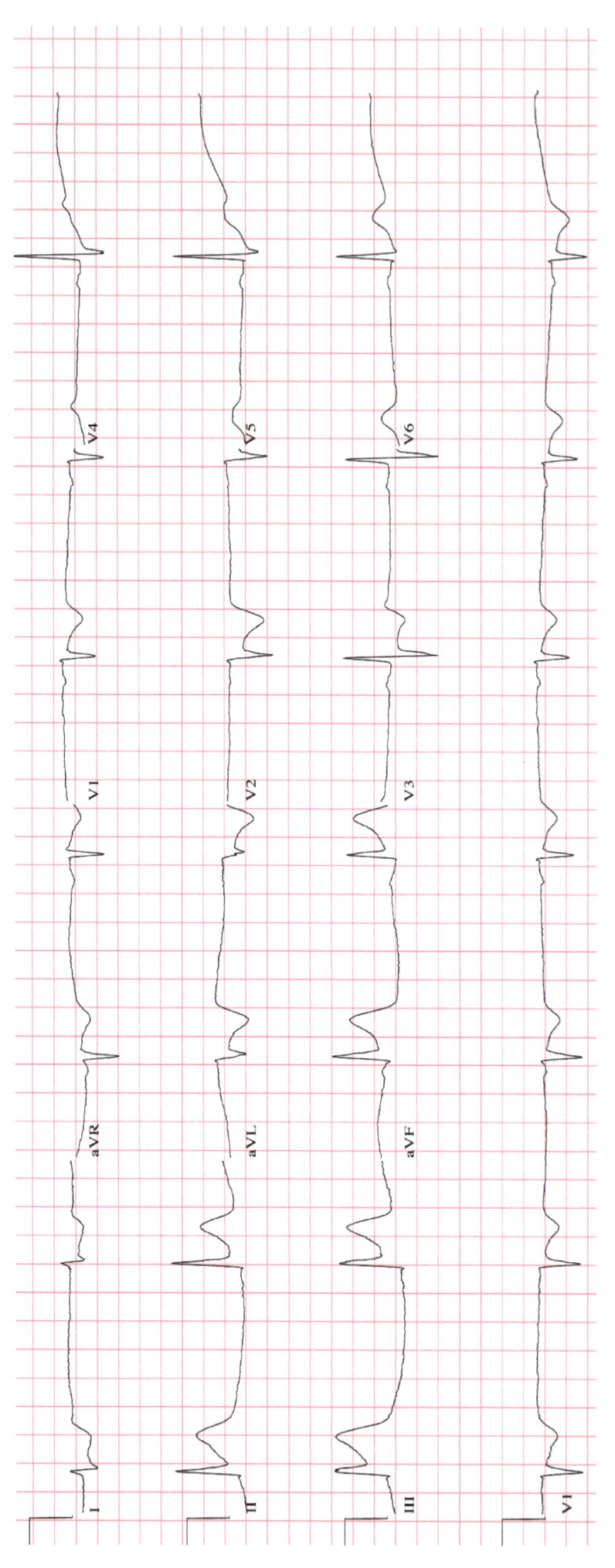

Infero-Posterior STEMI with sinus node dysfunction

Features:

- Inferior pattern- STE in II, III, aVF [12,48]
- RCA occlusion- STE in III > II and STD > 1 mm in lateral leads I and/or aVL (90% sensitive and 71% specific) [1,11,12,38,44] (See cases 6-7)
- Posterior pattern- STD in V_1-V_3 [44,48,56]

Clinical Pearls:

- High vagal tone during inferior Mis can cause reversible hypotension, bradycardia, AV block and junctional rhythms. [58] This is due to proximity to the fat pads that contain the vagal ganglions.
- In patients with bradycardia in inferior MI, consider administration of atropine to reverse bradycardia and place a temporary, rather than a permanent, pacemaker [51]

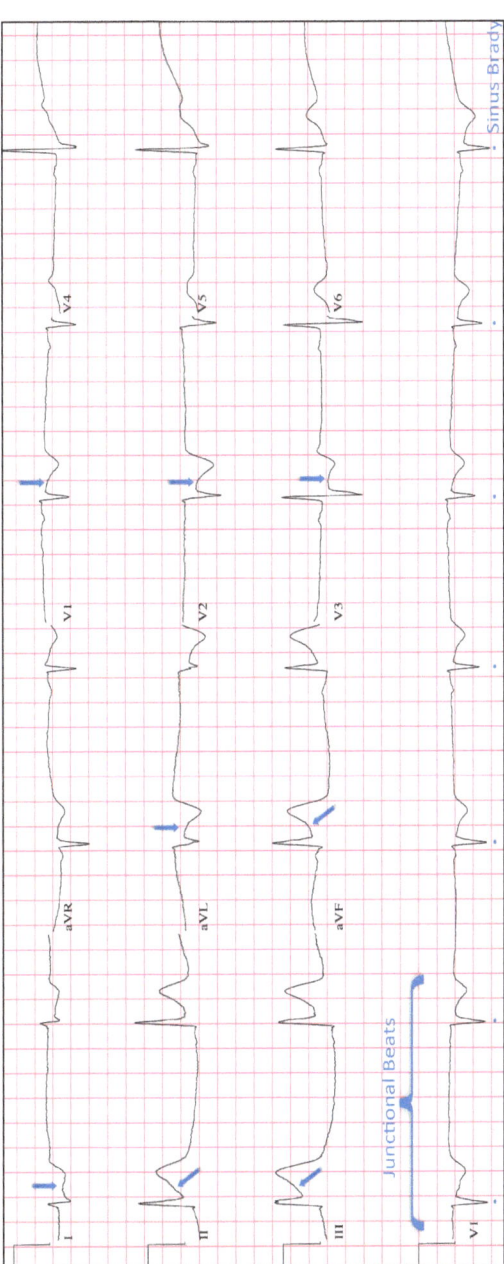

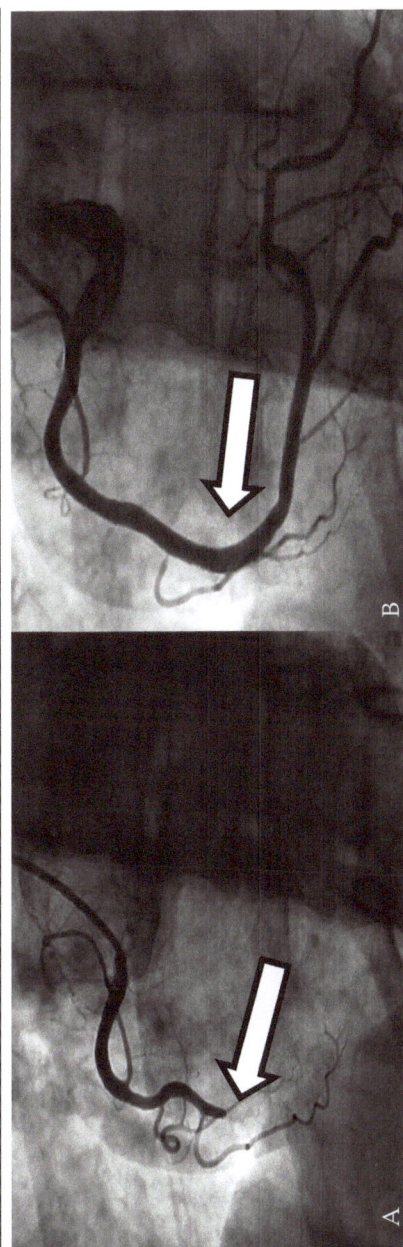

Fig. 13 A Pre-intervention cath image showing a 100% Mid-RCA occlusion (arrow). **B**, Post-intervention showing restored blood flow (arrow) supplying inferior, posterior and lateral myocardium.

NOTES

_____

_____

_____

Case 10: A 56 y.o. woman with HTN c/o squeezing chest pain 1 hour after cocaine use

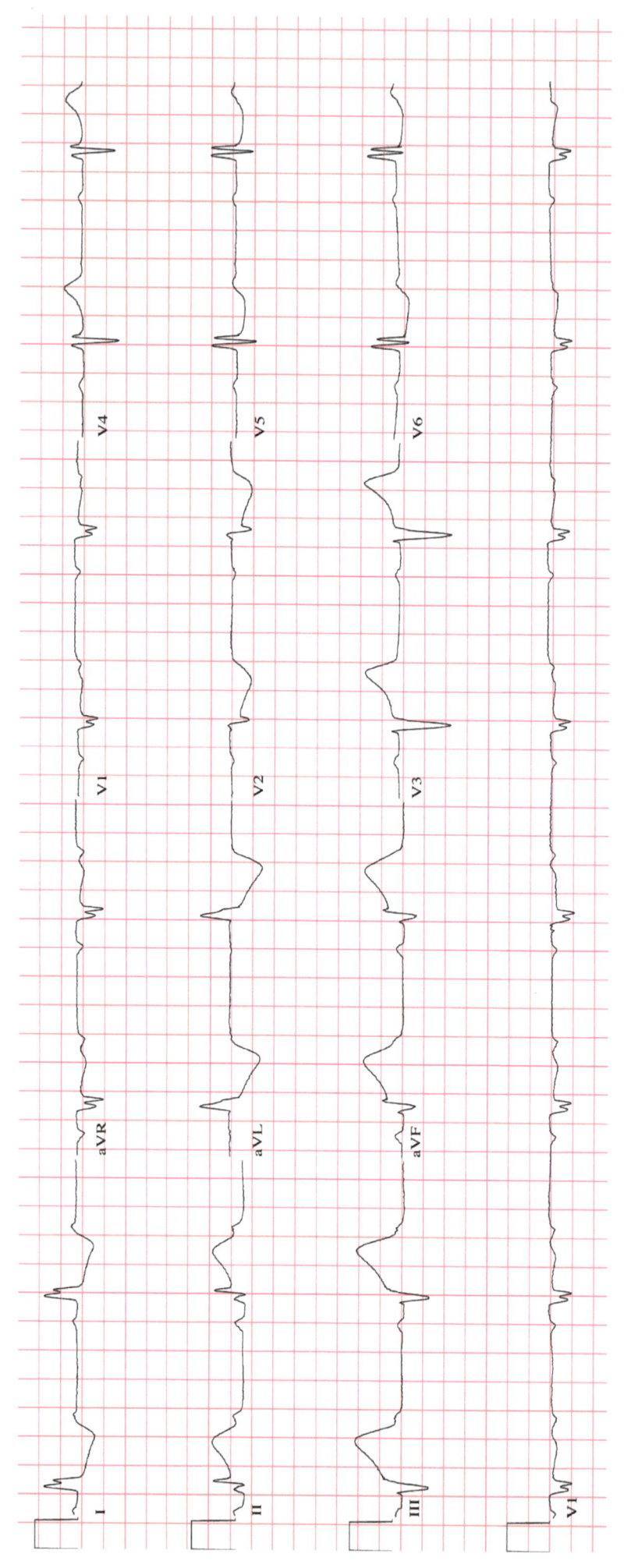

Infero-posterior STEMI with 2:1 AV Block

Features:

- Inferior pattern- STE in leads II, III, aVF[12,48]
  - RCA occlusion- STE in III > II and STD > 1 mm in lead I and/or aVL (Sensitivity 90%, Specificity 71%)[1,12,35,38,44]
- Posterior pattern- STD in V1-V$_2$[44,48,56]

Clinical Pearl:

- High vagal tone can cause bradycardia through it's effects on the AV node. Here we observe 2:1 AV block.
- Atropine may reverse bradycardia in high vagal tone scenario[58]
- If bradycardic, place a temporary rather than a permanent pacemaker because AV block may resolve[51]

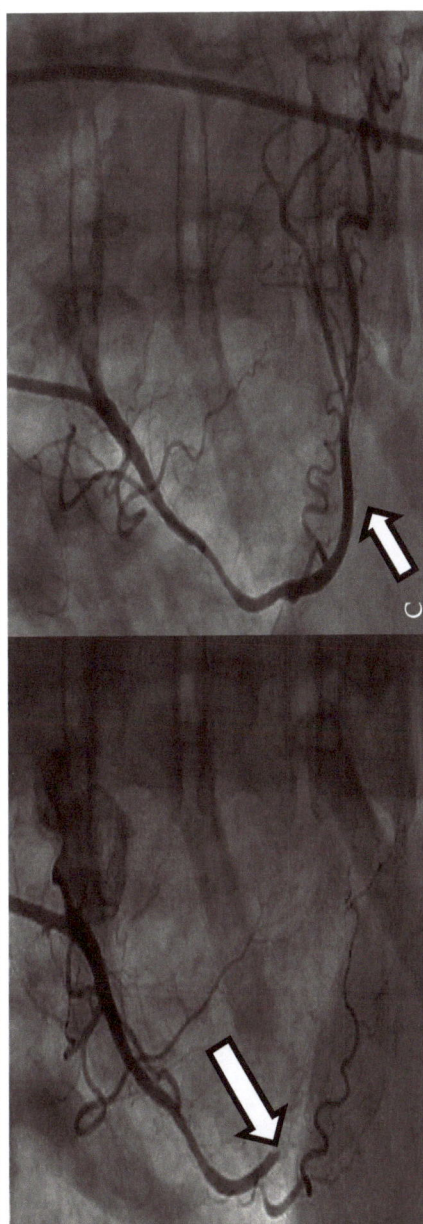

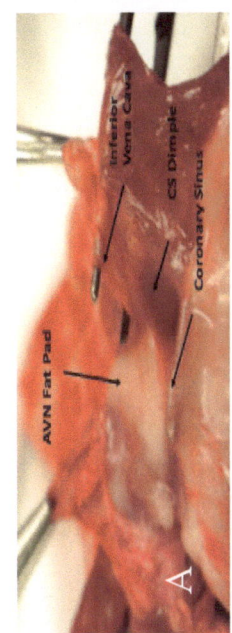

Fig. 14 A, A dissection of the AV Nodal fat pad, responsible for high vagal-tone. Note it's proximity to posterior cardiac structures, such as the coronary sinus and inferior vena cava. **B**, Pre-intervention cath image showing a 100% Mid-RCA occlusion (arrow). **C**, Post-intervention showing restored blood flow (arrow). Note this is a large caliber, dominant RCA.

35

Case 11: A 66 y.o. man c/o one hour of chest pressure a/w diaphoresis

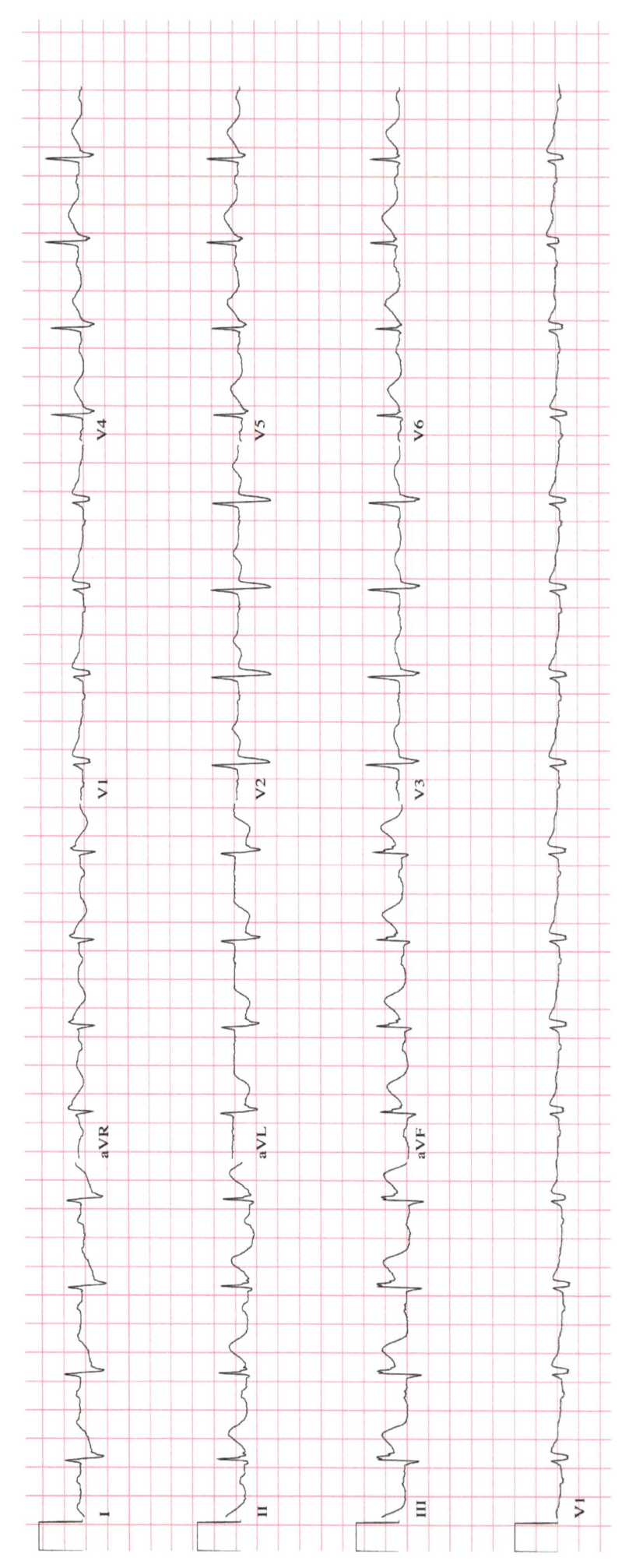

Infero-Posterior STEMI with Right Ventricular Infarction

Features:

- Inferior pattern- STE in II, III, aVF [12,48]
  - RCA occlusion- STE in III > II and STD > 1 mm in lead I and/or aVL (Sensitivity 90%, Specificity 71%)[1,11,12,38,44]
- Posterior pattern- STD in V_2, V_3 [44,48,56]
- Right ventricular infarction pattern- STE in V_1 and aVR (100% Specificity, 100% PPV) [1,38]

Other findings in this case:

- Lateral pattern- STD in I, aVL and STE in V_5, V_6 (indicates very dominant RCA)[13,48]
- Tall R-waves in V_2–V_3 are equivalent to Q-waves in the posterior wall [48,57]
- Small Q-waves in III and aVF indicate longer duration of ischemia

Clinical Pearl:

- Give IV fluids in RV infarct to maintain pre-load. These patients are pre-load dependent. Do NOT give nitroglycerin because it decreases pre-load [51]

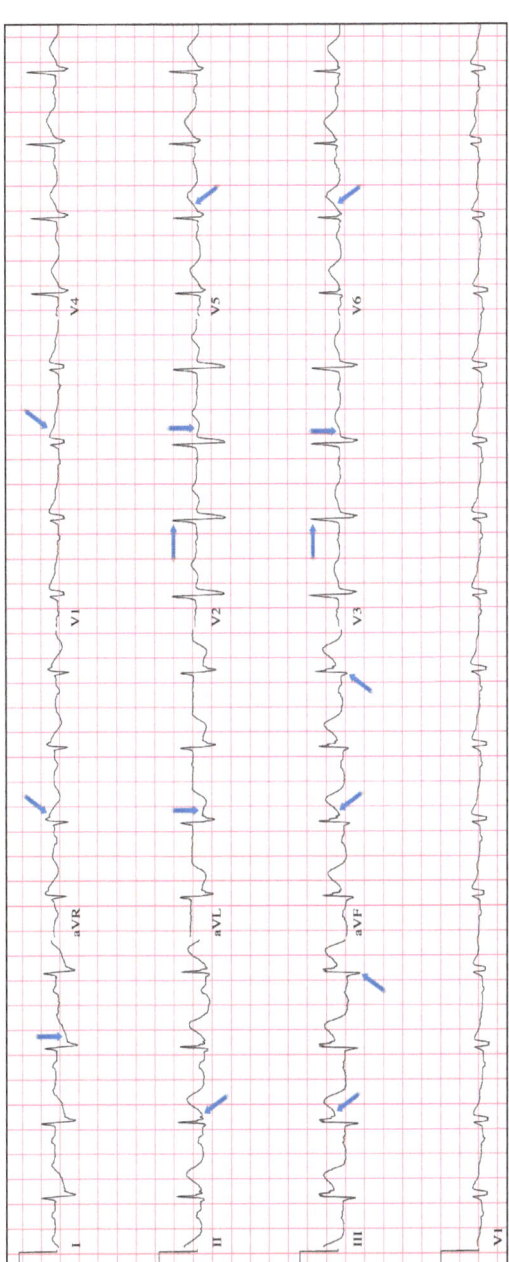

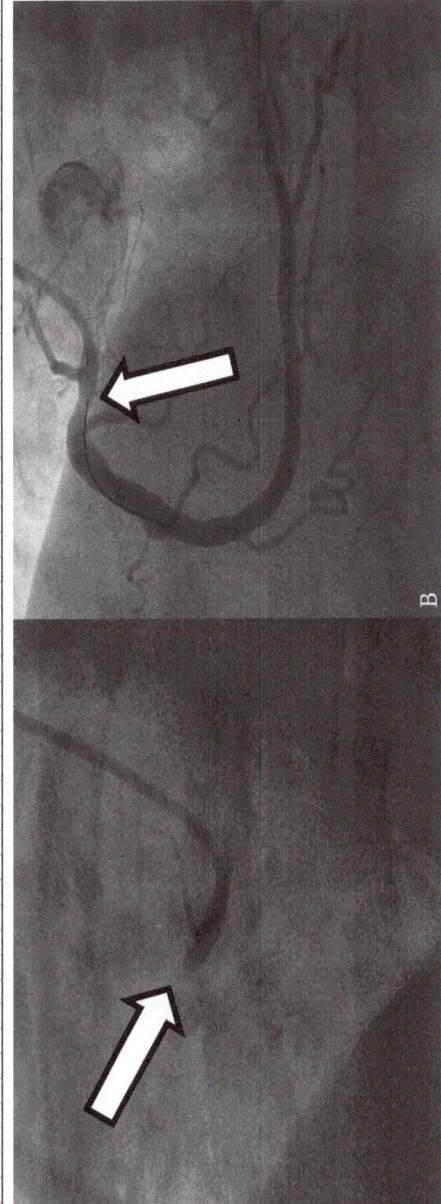

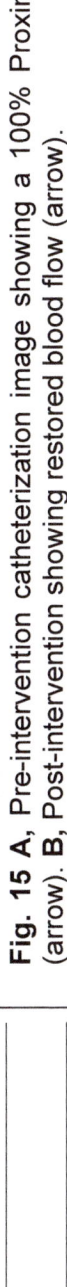

Fig. 15 A, Pre-intervention catheterization image showing a 100% Proximal RCA occlusion (arrow). **B,** Post-intervention showing restored blood flow (arrow).

<u>NOTES</u>

Case 12: A 62 y.o. man with HTN and HLD c/o 10 hours of constant chest pain

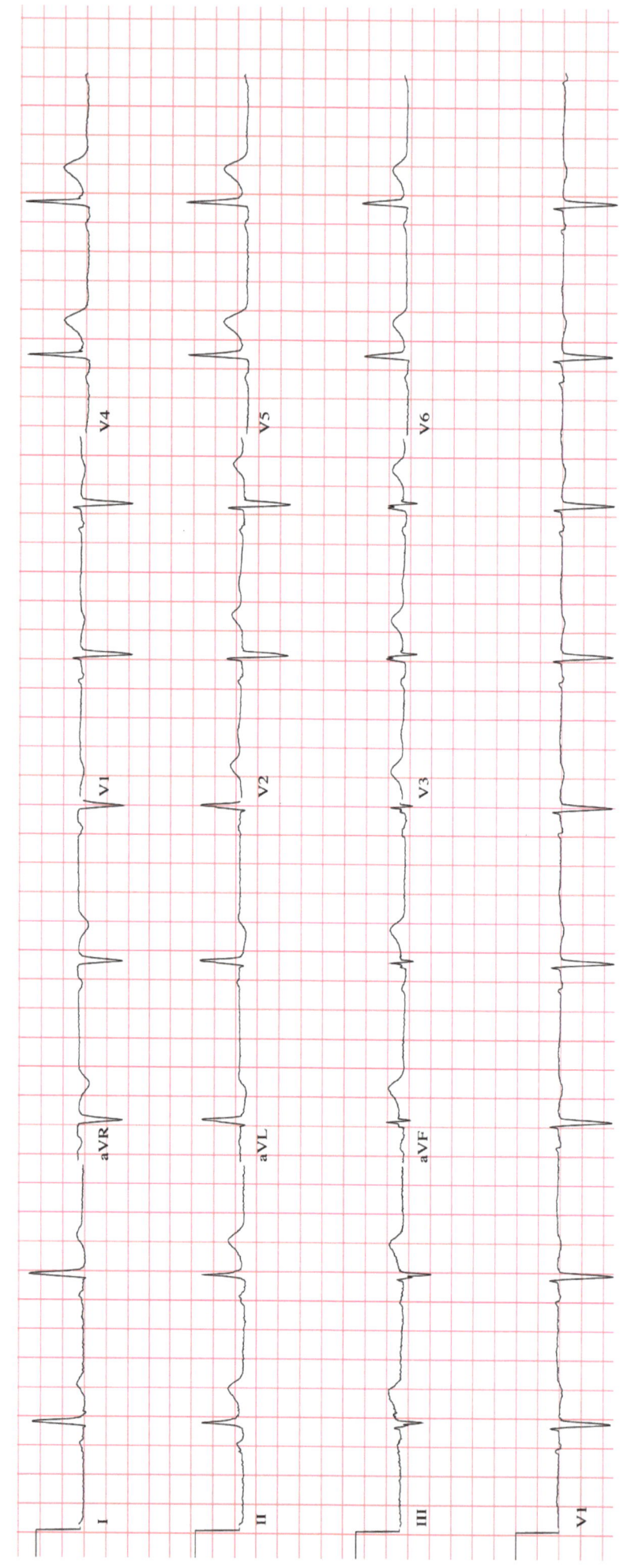

Lateral STEMI

Features:
- Lateral pattern- STE in V_4-V_6 [13,42,60]
- LCx System Occlusion- STD in aVL [13,48]

Other findings in this case:
- Small amount of STE in II, III, aVF indicate some inferior wall involvement [12]
- There is a large circumflex system in this case. Note the large caliber circumflex vessels and flow through the OM3 and its branches towards the apex.

Clinical Pearls:
- The circumflex territory is considered to be somewhat electrically silent. The EKG manifestations of ischemia and infarction can therefore be overlooked given their subtlety. In this case, a total occlusion of the large-caliber OM3 system causes fairly subtle EKG changes. Compare this to anterior infarctions, where EKG manifestations are more dramatic. This also underscores the importance of taking the clinical presentation into consideration when deciding whether to activate the catheterization lab.

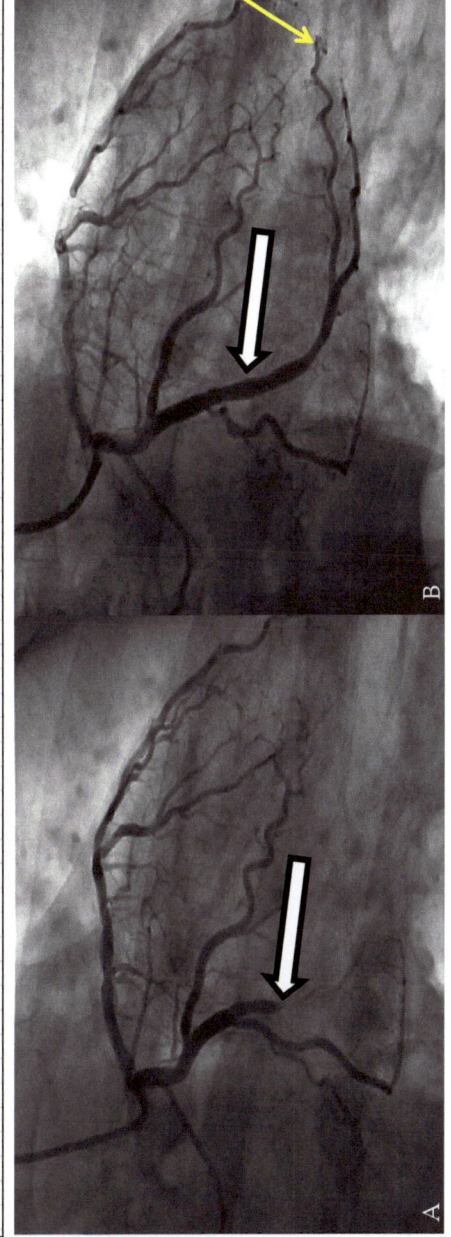

Fig. 16 A, Pre-intervention catheterization image showing a 100% OM occlusion (arrow). **B,** Post-intervention showing restored blood flow (yellow arrow).

NOTES
_____

39

STEMI EQUIVALENTS

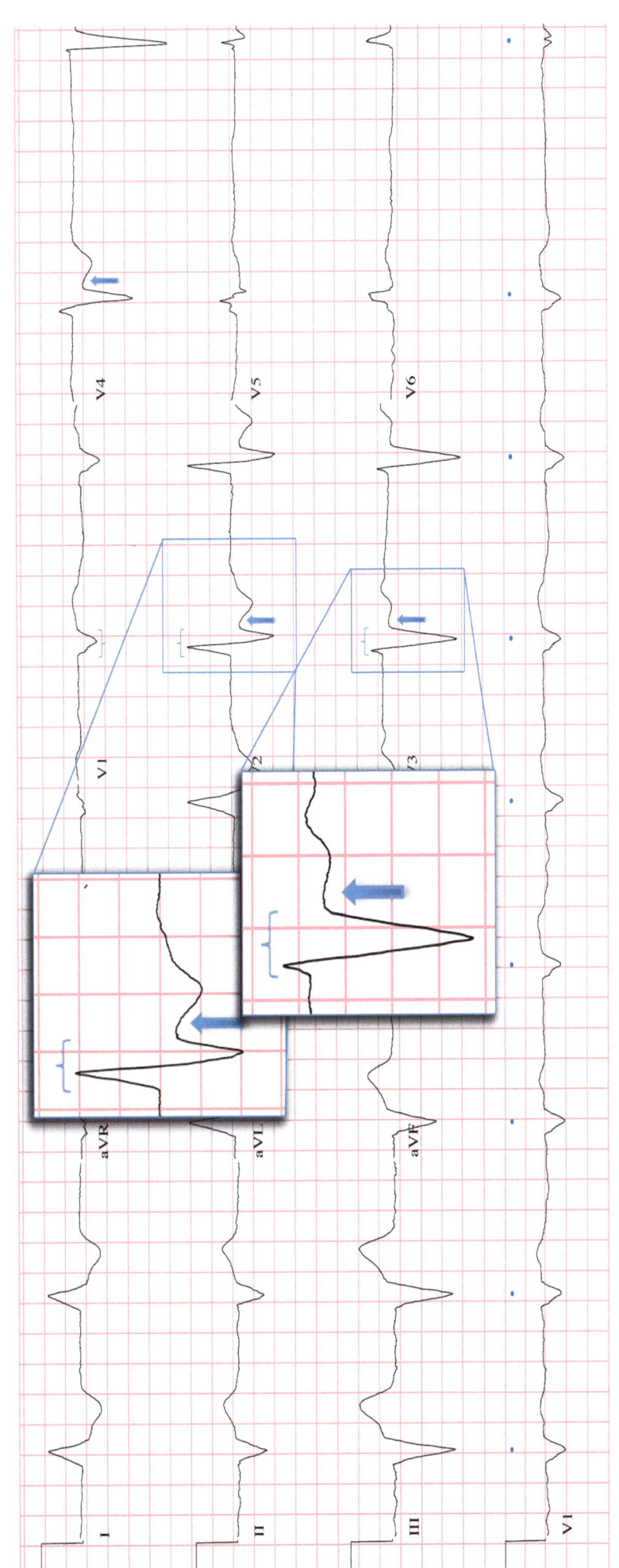

Case 13: A 69 y.o. man with CAD, DM, HTN, and HLD c/o chest pain

STEMI with Existing LBBB

Features:

- LBBB pattern:[1,48,61]
  - Wide QRS > 120ms
  - Notched R-wave in I, aVL, V$_5$, V$_6$ (note this can be subtle)
  - Discordant deviation of ST-segments and T-waves relative to orientation of QRS complex
- Sgarbossa criteria- Used to diagnose MI when LBBB present:
  - Concordant STE in a lead with a positive QRS ≥ 1 mm (5 pts)
  - STD ≥ 1mm in V$_1$–V$_3$ (3 pts)
  - Discordant STE in a lead with a negative QRS ≥ 5mm (2pts)

≥ 3 points- 90% specificity for MI[16,17,38, 62, 63]

Other findings in this case:
- Atrial fibrillation
- STD in V$_1$–V$_3$ indicate posterior involvement due to dominant LCx artery perfusing a large territory (smaller arrow)

QRS>120ms

Atrial Fibrillation

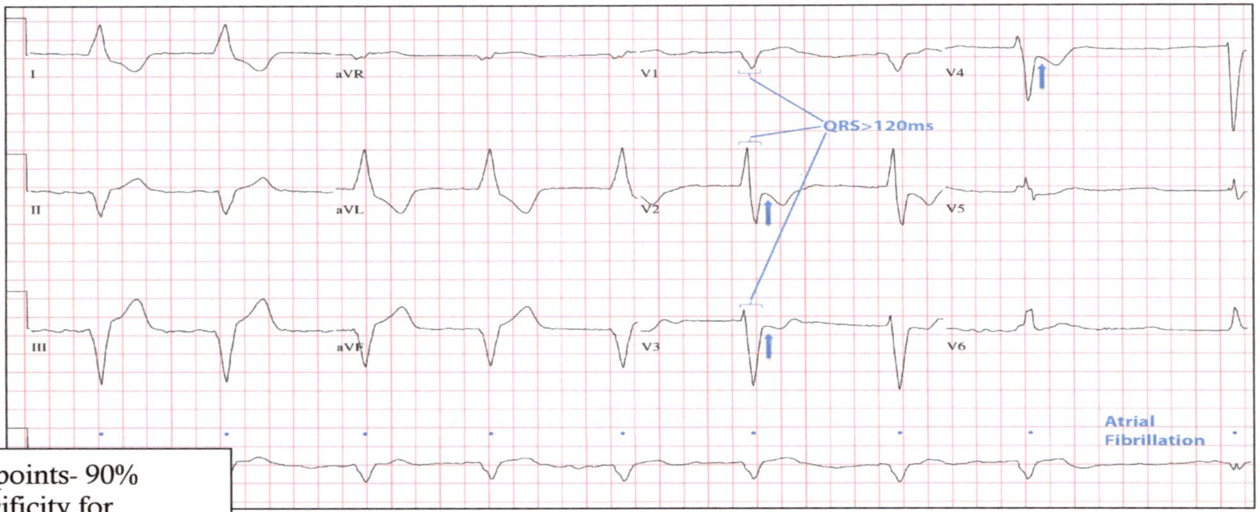

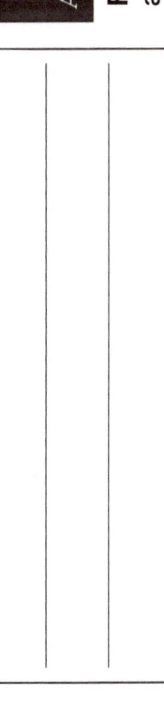

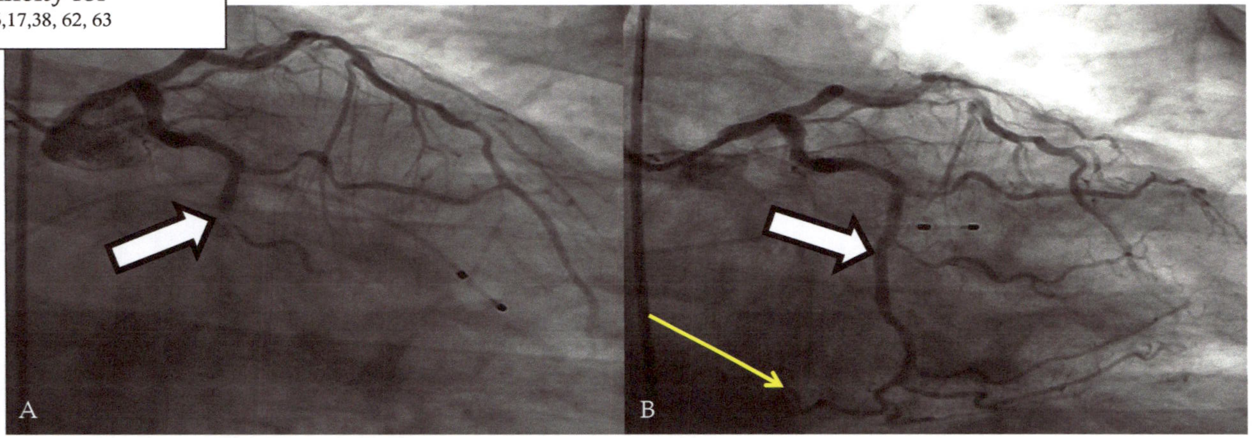

Fig. 17 A, Pre-intervention image, 100% LCx occlusion (arrow). **B,** Restored blood flow (large arrow) showing a dominant LCx supplying lateral and posterior wall (yellow arrow).

NOTES

Case 14: A 44 y.o. man with HTN, DM, and HLD c/o chest pain that began while gardening

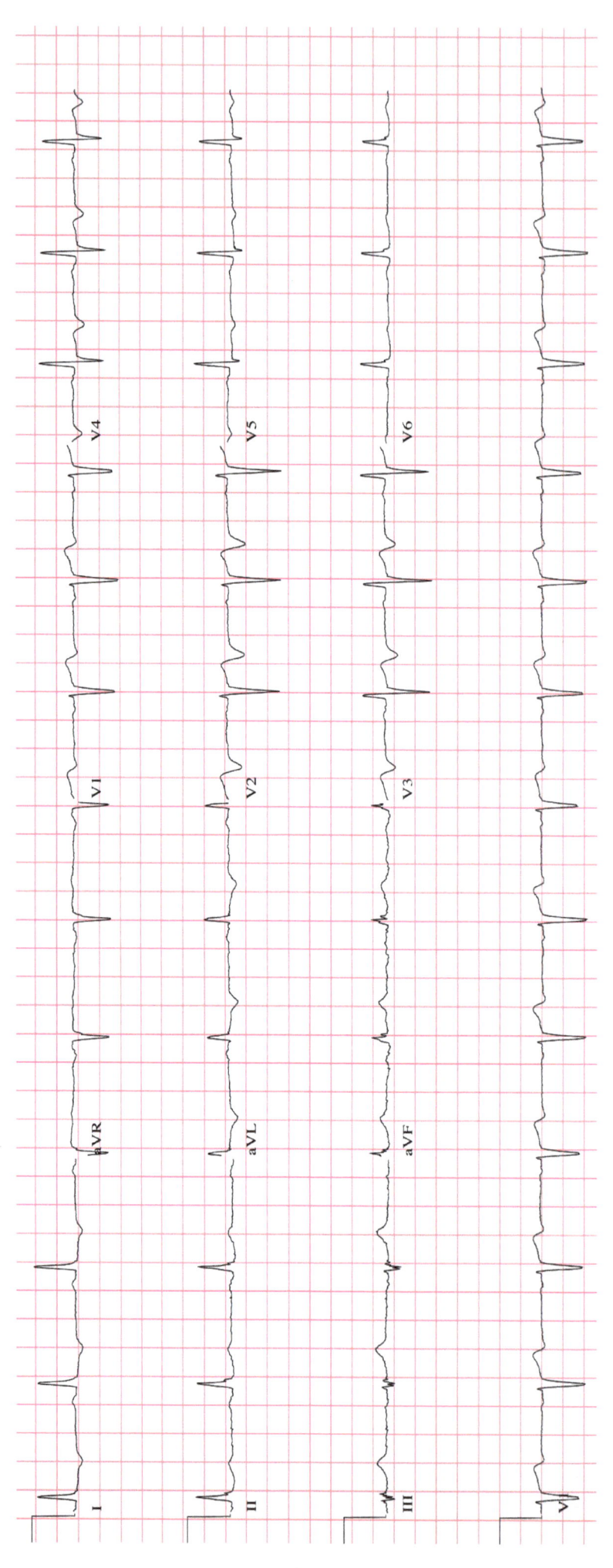

Wellens' Syndrome

Features:

- Biphasic or inverted T-waves in V_2, V_3
  - Note in this case the T-wave changes extend out to V_5 in a diminishing fashion
- Negative or minimally elevated cardiac biomarkers[65]

Clinical Pearls:

- Wellens' Syndrome indicates high-degree stenosis of the proximal LAD and an impending anterior STEMI[23]
- It is an indication for urgent catheterization and no stress test should be done! [65,66,67]

NOTES

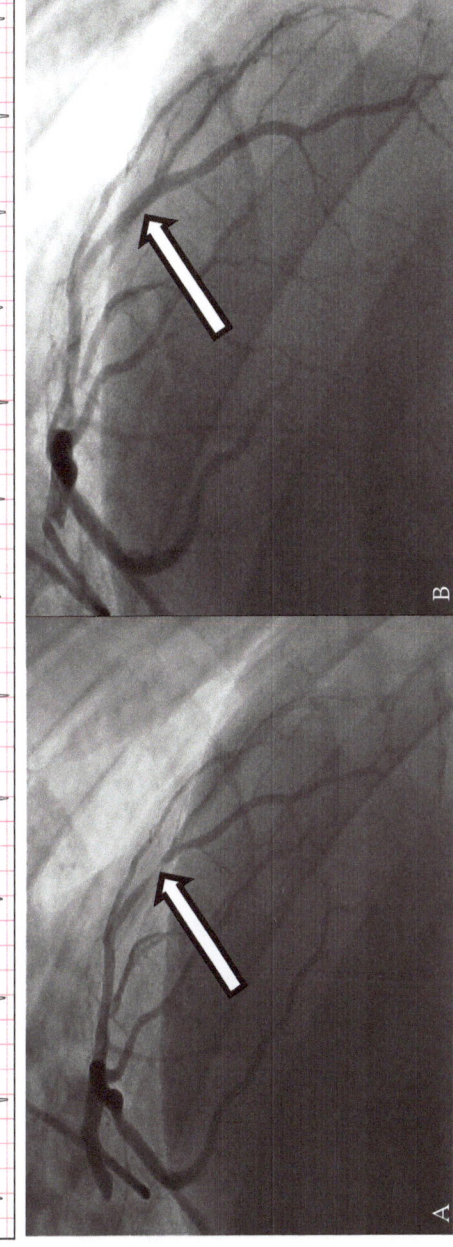

Fig. 18 A, Pre-intervention cath image showing a 99% stenosis in the Mid-LAD (arrow). Note there is some distal blood flow **B,** Post-intervention showing restored blood flow (arrow).

Case 15: A 56 y.o. man with IVDA and HIV presents to the ER with chest pain

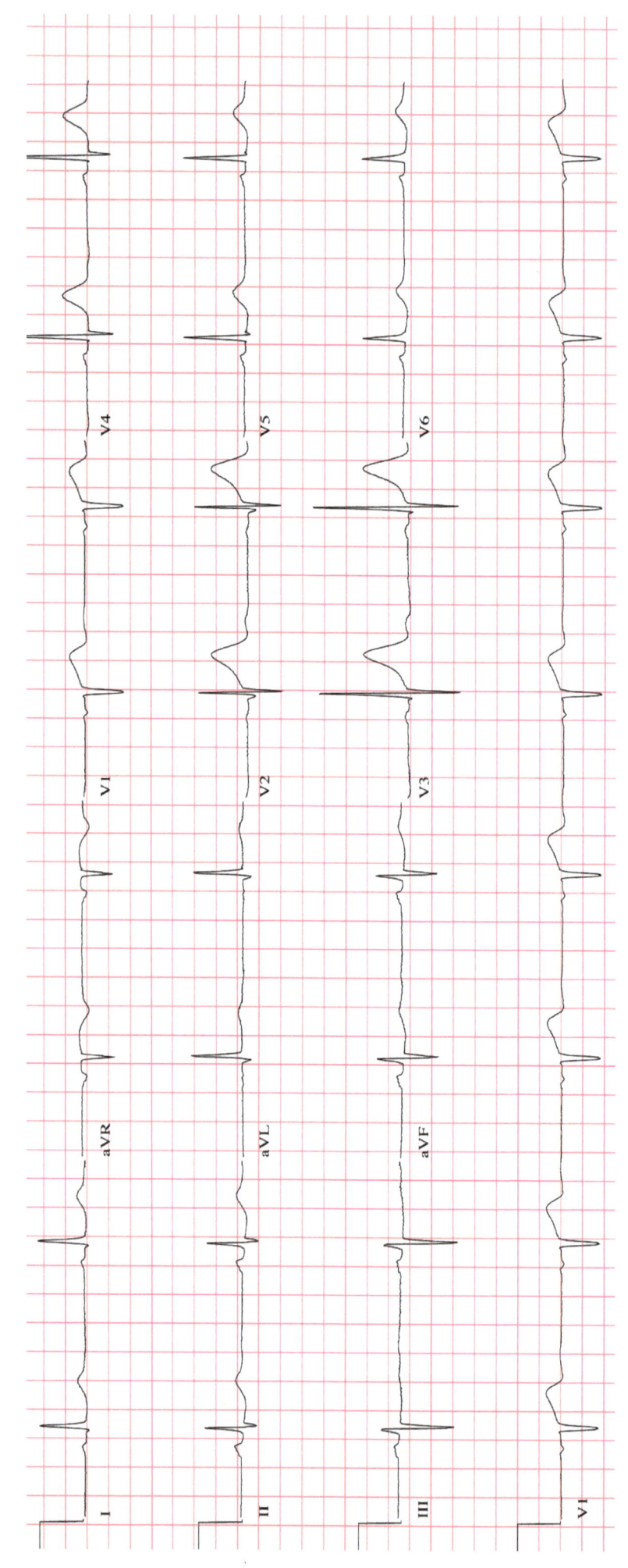

Hyperacute T-Waves

Features:

- Tall prominent, although not necessarily peaked, T-waves in V_2-V_3 that occur within minutes of an acute coronary occlusion
- Quickly change to a classic STEMI pattern[24,64,68,69]
- Notice minimal STE in anterior leads and minor changes in the slope of ST segment
- Loss of concavity of ST segment in V_1 when compared to other anterior leads will become marked and spread with time
- Inferior wall involvement: Reciprocal STD in leads II, III, aVF

Clinical Pearl:
Repeat EKG in 10 minutes and it will likely show typical STEMI pattern

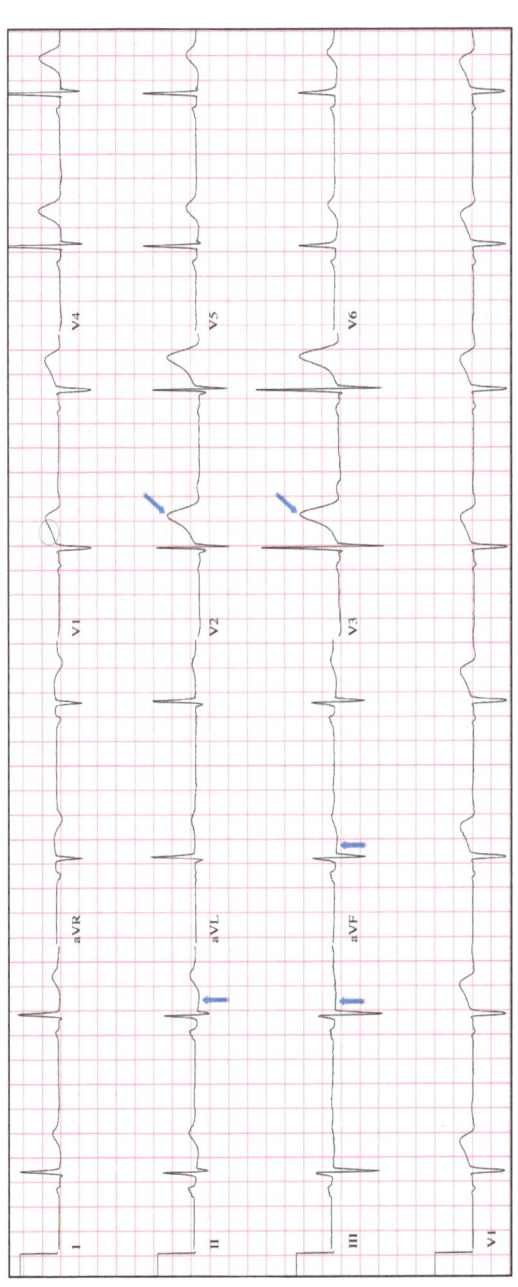

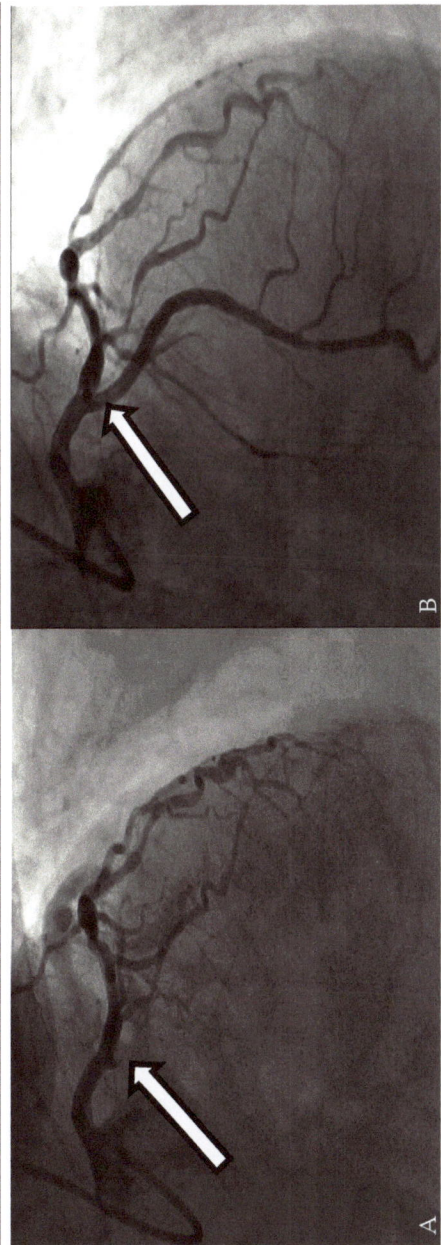

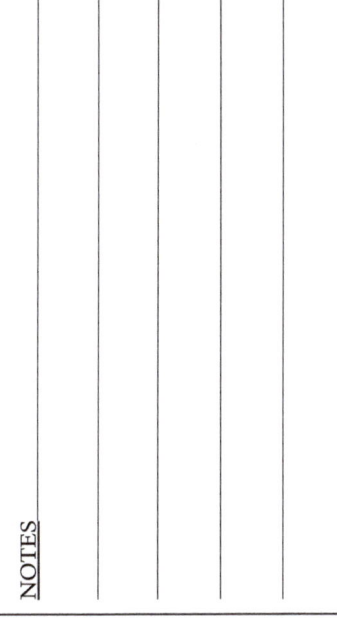

Fig. 19 A, Pre-intervention catheterization image showing a 100% LAD occlusion (arrow). **B,** Post-intervention showing restored blood flow (arrow).

NOTES

STEMI Mimics

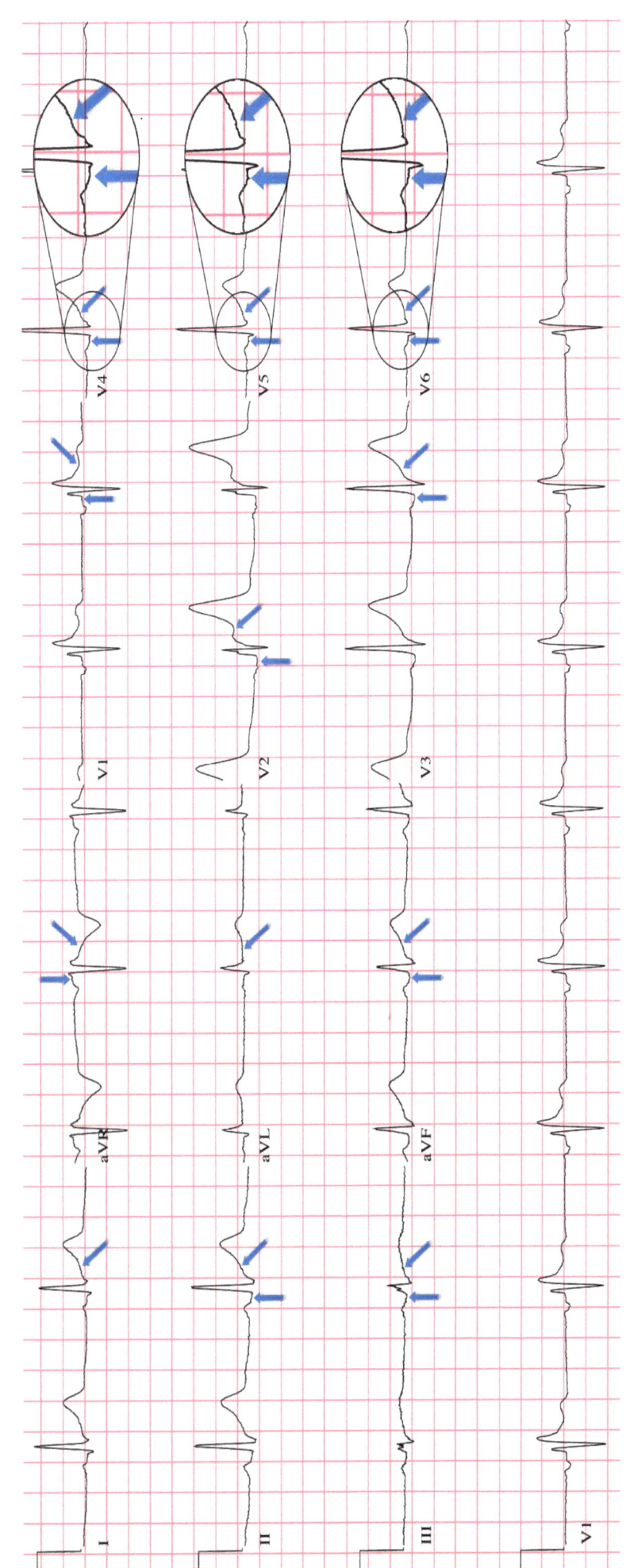

Case 16: A 79 y.o. man s/p infero-lateral STEMI and known LBBB c/o atypical chest pain

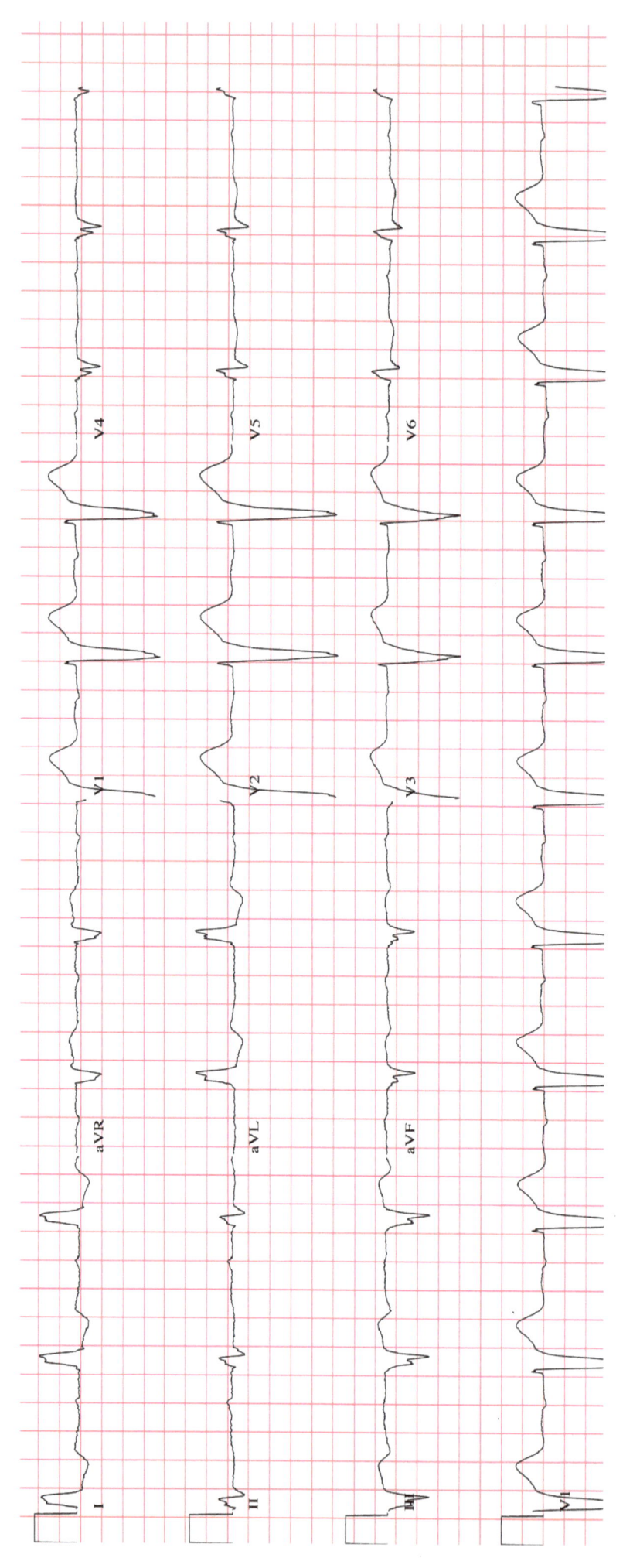

Left Bundle Branch Block

Features:

- LBBB-
  - Wide QRS > 120ms
  - Notched R-wave in I, aVL, V_5, V_6
  - Discordant deviation of ST-segments and T-waves relative to orientation of QRS complex[48,61,70]

Clinical Pearls:

- Given LBBB is associated with STE in anterior leads, it is often brings STEMI to mind. The first step in determining if AMI is present is to obtain a prior EKG to determine if the LBBB is pre-existing. A new LBBB in the setting of very convincing, typical chest pain is a STEMI-equivalent and merits activating the catheterization lab. If no EKG is available, the clinical history and Sgarbossa criteria are used to determine if an AMI is present (see Case 13)

Other finding in this case:

- Q waves and notched QRS pattern seen along inferior leads c/w prior infarction of that area

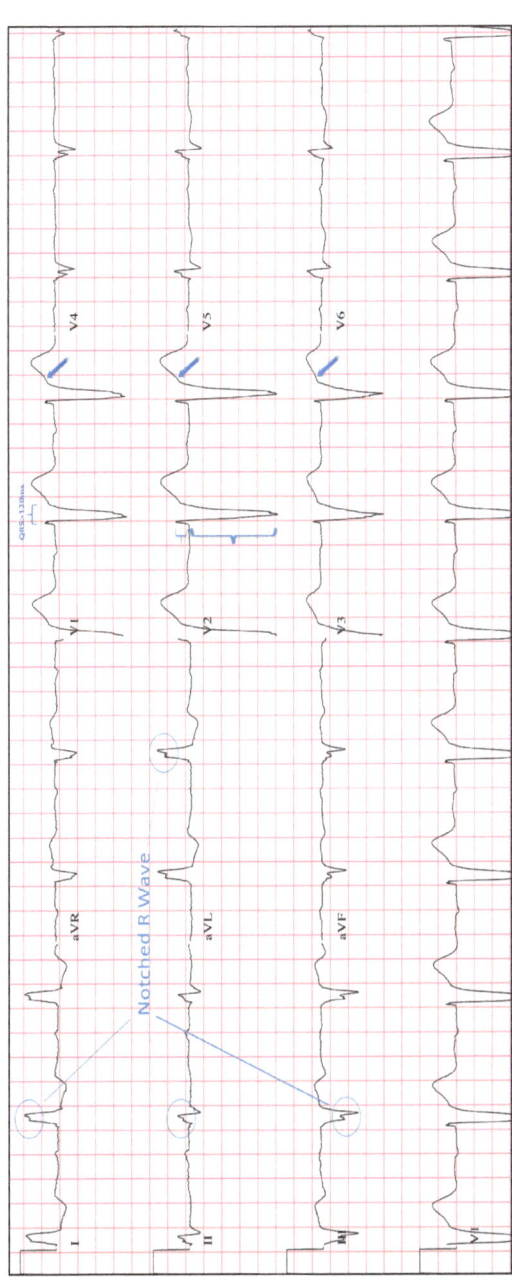

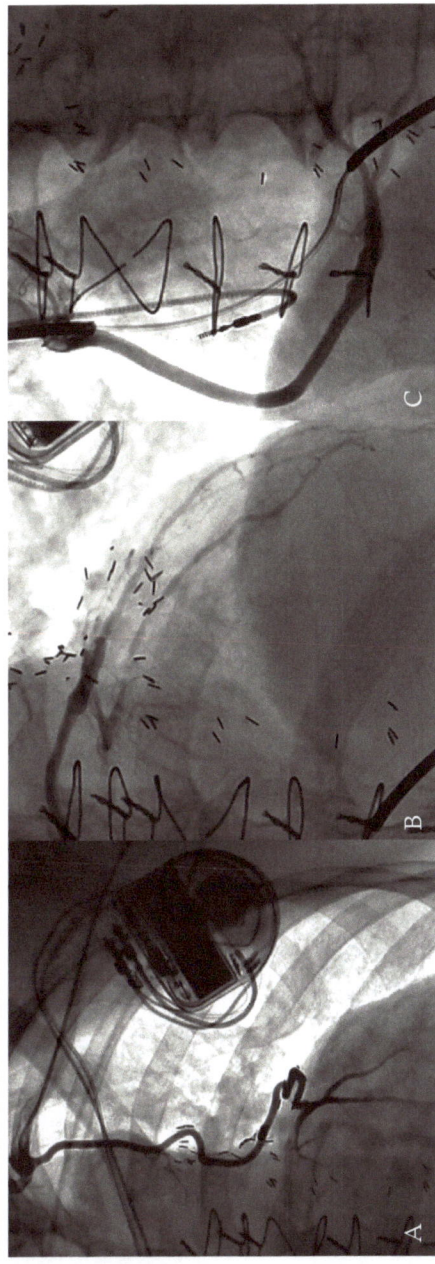

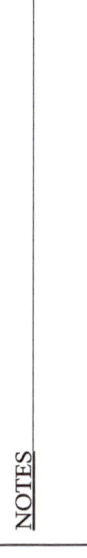

Fig. 20 Cath images showing chronic total occlusion of the left main with patent LIMA to LAD graft (**A**) and patent SVG-to-OM (**B**), and SVG-to-RCA (**C**) grafts.

<u>NOTES</u>

Case 17: A 54 y.o. man c/o two days of intermittent pleuritic chest pain which woke him from sleep

Pericarditis

Features:

- Diffuse STE and PR depressions with PR elevation and STD in aVR[28,71,72,73]

- Maintenance of STE concavity is typical. Compare the shape of ST-segments in this case to the tombstoning of the classic anterior MIs (See cases 2 & 3)

- Diffuse J-point elevation seen early, as in this case, but can later normalize and be followed by TWI[74]

Clinical Pearls:

- Patient history is important to make diagnosis

- Look for pleuritic pain with mono-, bi-, or tri-phasic rub on auscultation

- Colchicine, when added to conventional anti-inflammatory therapy (ibuprofen or aspirin), significantly reduces the rate of recurrent pericarditis[59]

<u>NOTES</u>

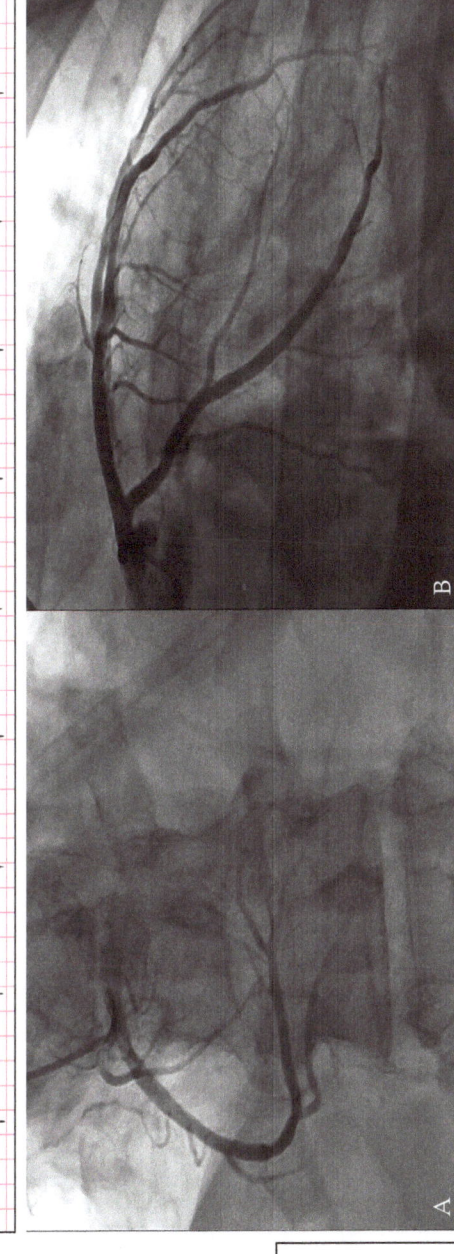

Fig. 21 Catheterization images showing patent RCA (**A**), LAD and LCx systems (**B**).

53

Case 18: A 50 y.o. man h/o antero-lateral STEMI and CHF (EF 13%), shocked 3 times by his defibrillator

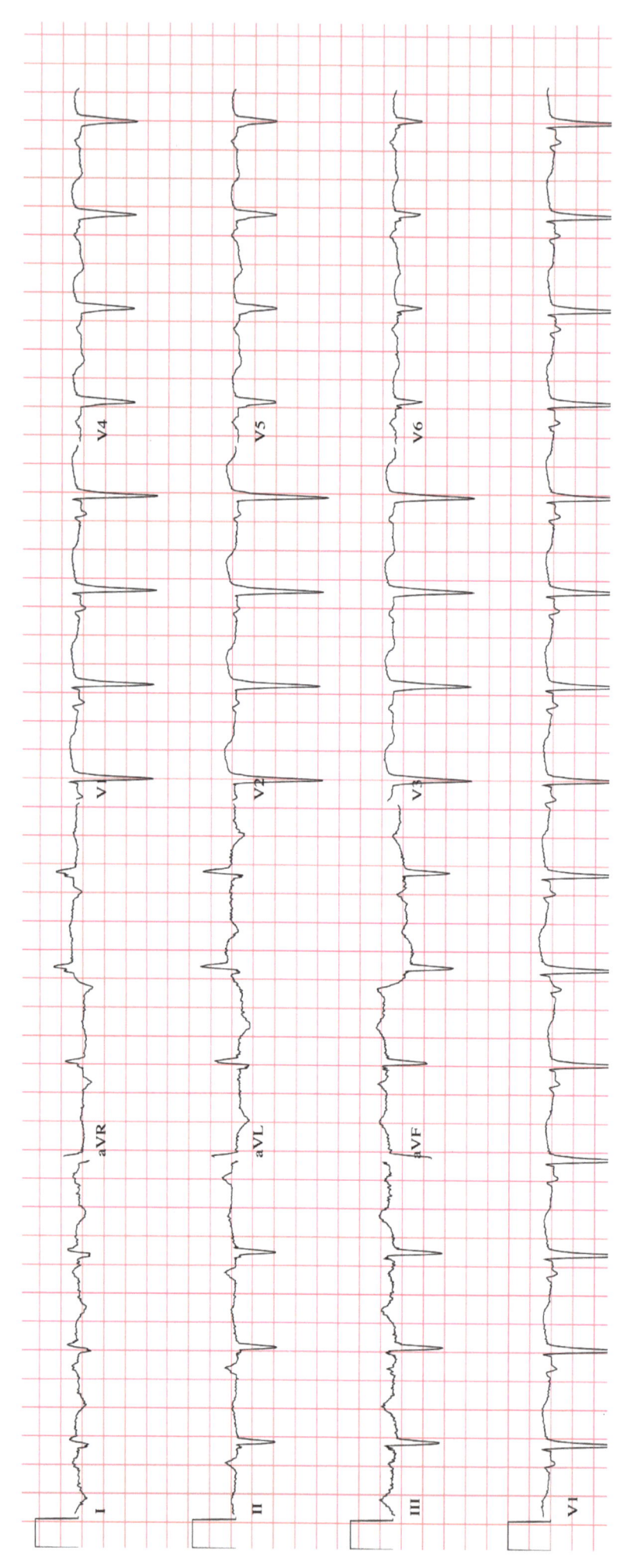

Ventricular Aneurysm

Features:
- Persistent STE in V_1-V_3 with pathologic Q-waves in a patient with history of MI[48,75,76]
  - Typical for left ventricular aneurysm

Other findings in this case:
- T-wave inversions are noted in leads I, aVL, V_3-V_5[76]
- Echo results (Fig. 22A): Dilated left ventricle. Left ventricular apex appears aneurysmal (arrows). Segmental left ventricular wall motion abnormalities. (Fig. 22B): Normal LV for comparison

Clinical Pearls:
- Note the absence of chest pain in the history. These patients will present for follow up evaluations and be found to have an EKG that looks like a STEMI. Comparison to a prior EKG is essential and should confirm that the ST elevations have been present in the past.

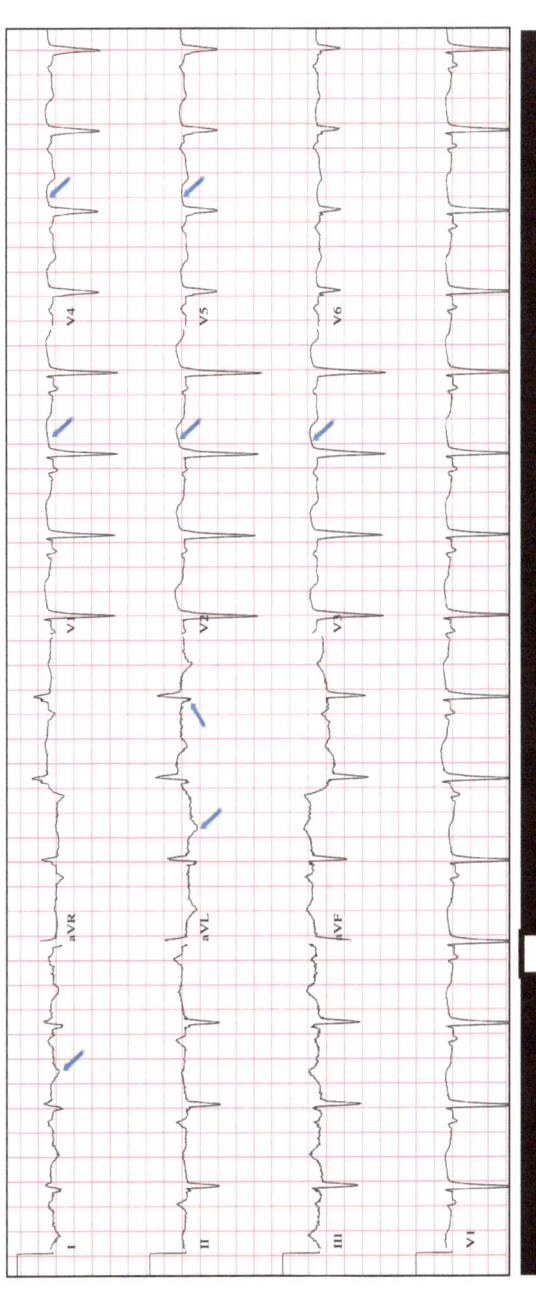

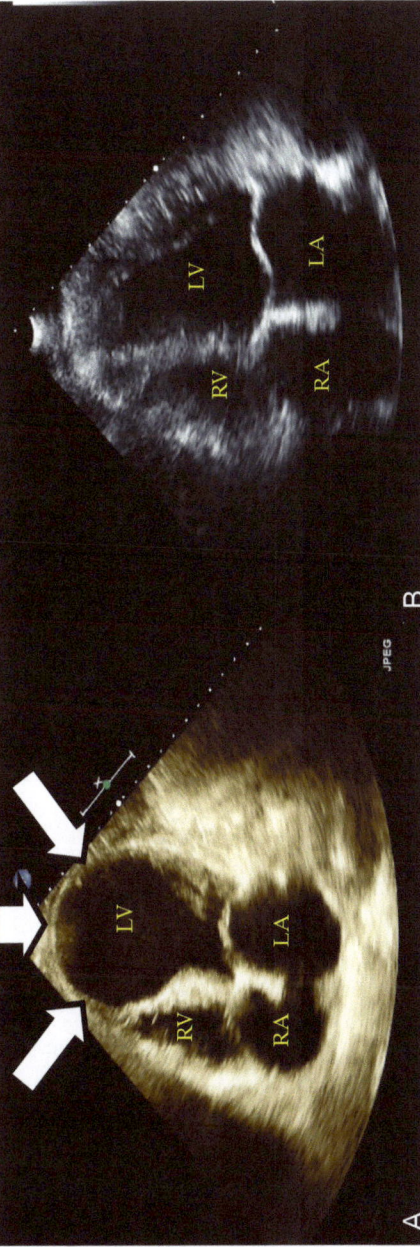

Fig. 22 Echocardiogram images showing aneurysmal apex of the LV in systole (**A**) as compared to a normal LV in systole (**B**).

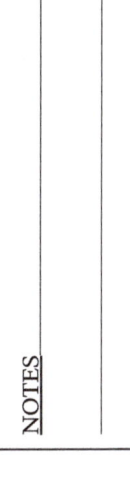

NOTES

Case 19: A 75 y.o. man with HLD and COPD c/o 3 days of chest pressure and dyspnea a/w troponin of 5

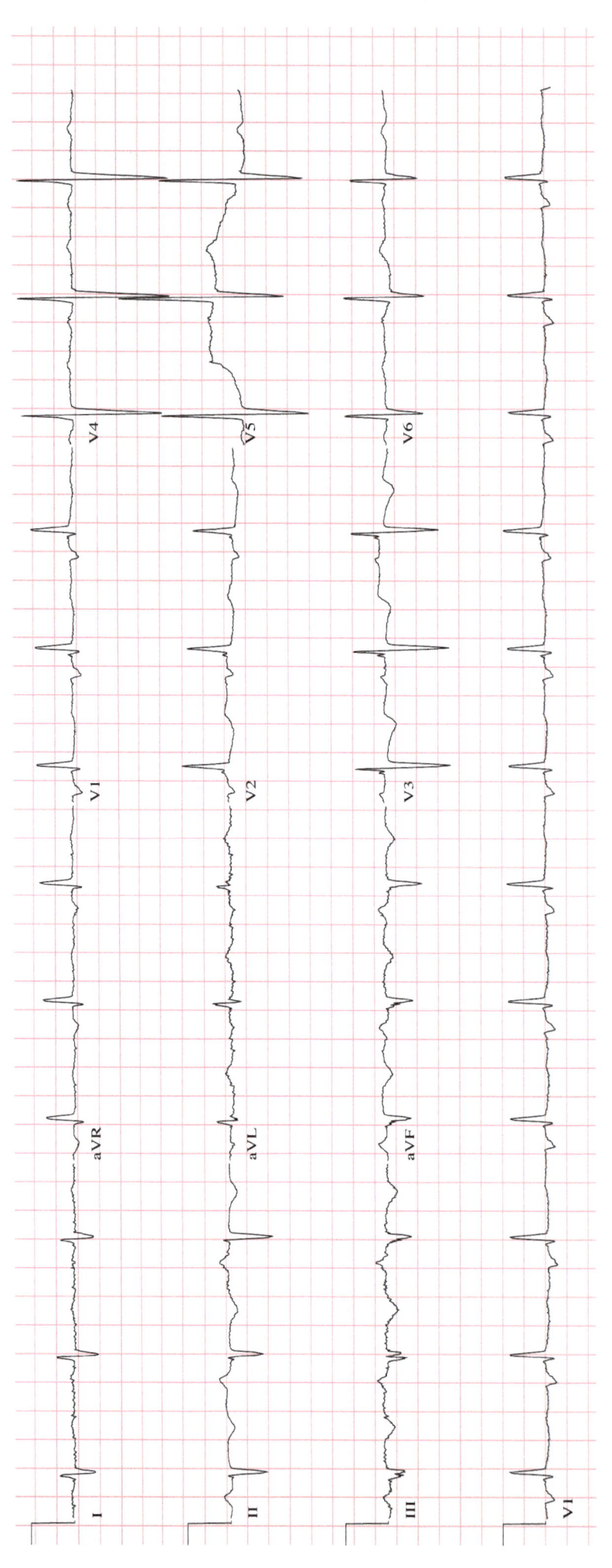

Pulmonary Embolism

Features:

- $S_IQ_{III}T_{III}$ (S-wave in lead I, Q-wave and inverted T-wave in lead III) – The "classic" EKG finding seen in only 20% of pulmonary embolism. It is a manifestation of acute pressure and volume overload of the right ventricle [36,51,77,78]

- Right Heart Strain – T wave inversions in the right precordial leads (V1-V3) and the inferior leads (II, III aVL) [36,51,78]

Other EKG changes

- RSR' in V_1, V_2 and aVL
- Pseudonormalization in V_1, aVL (see cases 4 & 5)
- Lateralization of the QRS transition from negative to positive from V_3 to V_5

Clinical Pearl

- The positive troponin is due to right heart pressure overload and does not mean myocardial infarction! [51]

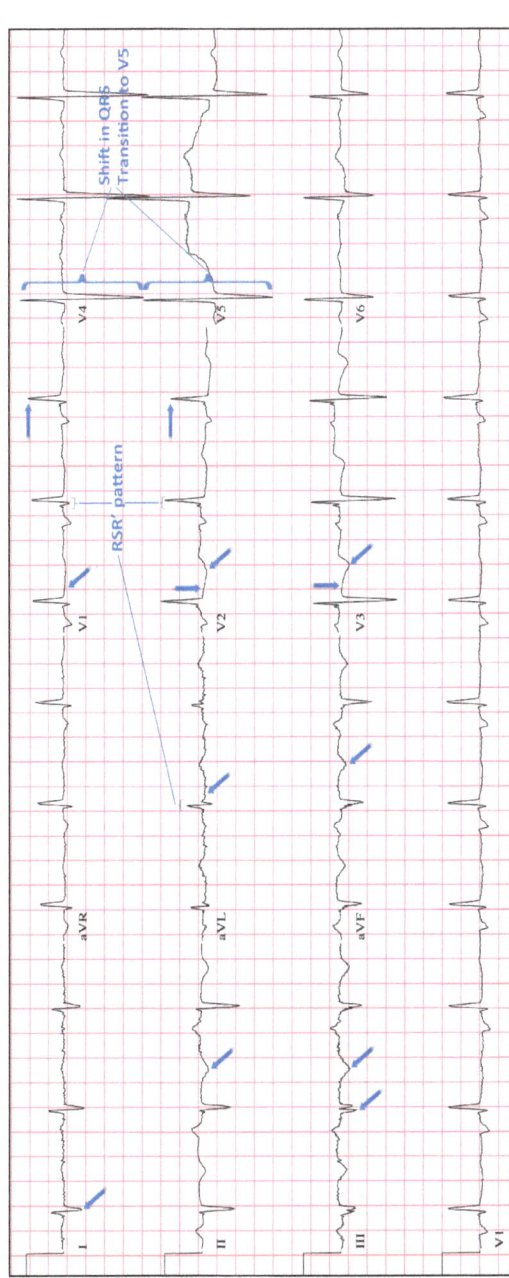

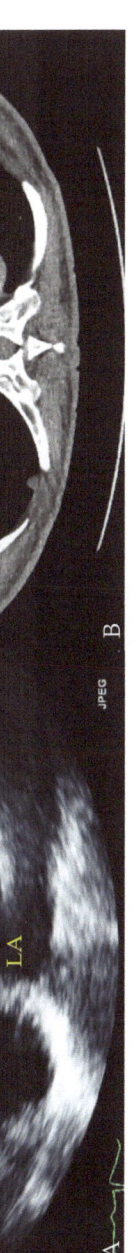

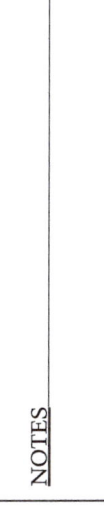

Fig. 23 A, An apical 4-Chamber Echocardiogram image showing enlarged RV and RA. **B,** CT-Angiogram image showing extensive bilateral acute and chronic pulmonary emboli (arrows).

<u>NOTES</u>

Case 20: A 41 y.o. woman with HTN, DM, and a normal angiogram c/o substernal chest pressure

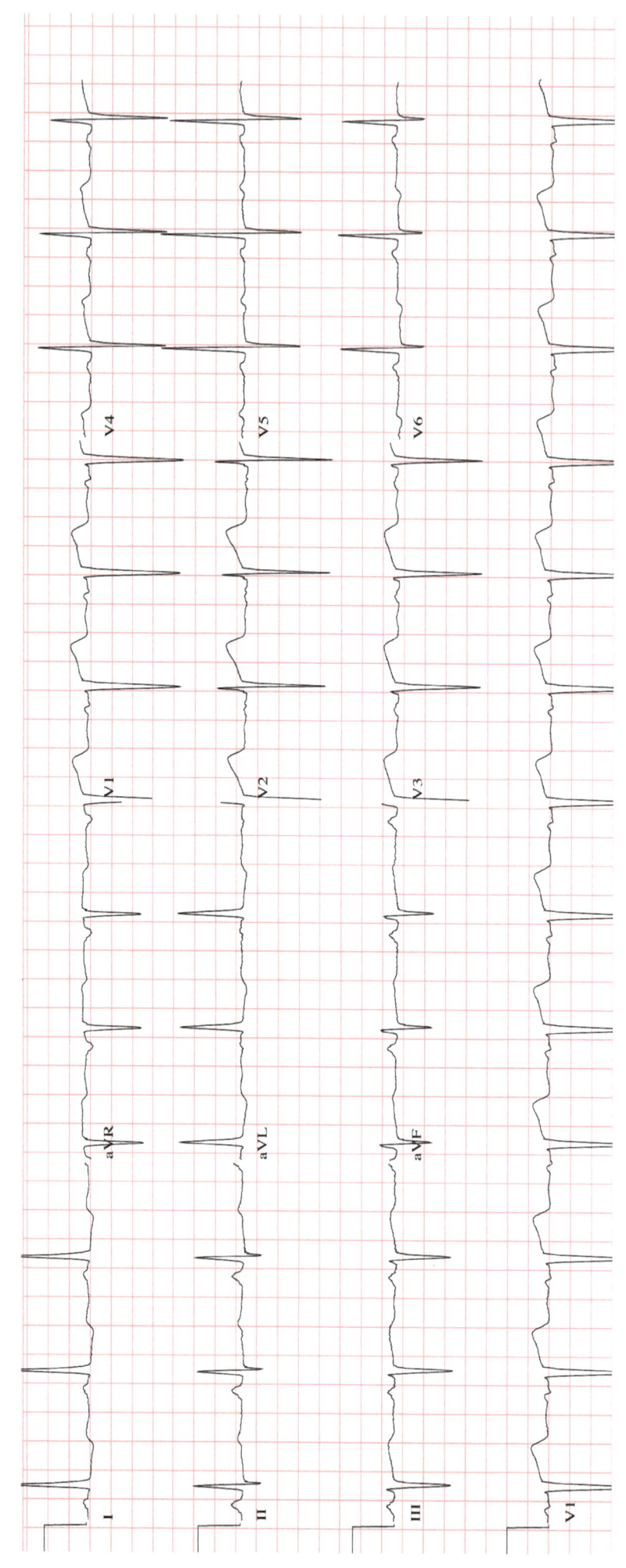

Left Ventricular Hypertrophy

Features:

- Cornell Criteria (specificity 98%)- S-wave in V_3 + R-wave in aVL >28mm in men, >20mm in women[33,79,80]

- Sokolow-Lyon Index- S-wave in V_1 + tallest R-wave height in V_5 or V_6 > 35 mm[32,48]

- ST and T-wave abnormalities can be seen because of repolarization abnormalities in anterior and lateral leads. These do not represent ischemia![48]

Clinical Pearl:

- There are many EKG criteria that can be used to diagnose LVH. The above two are the most sensitive and specific and therefore, the most commonly used.

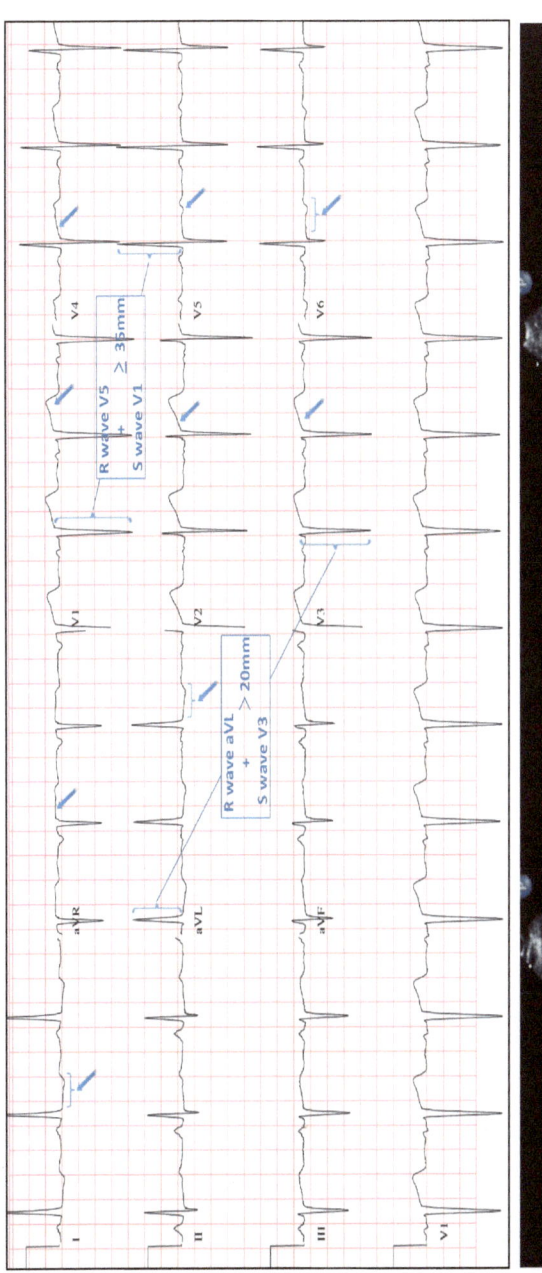

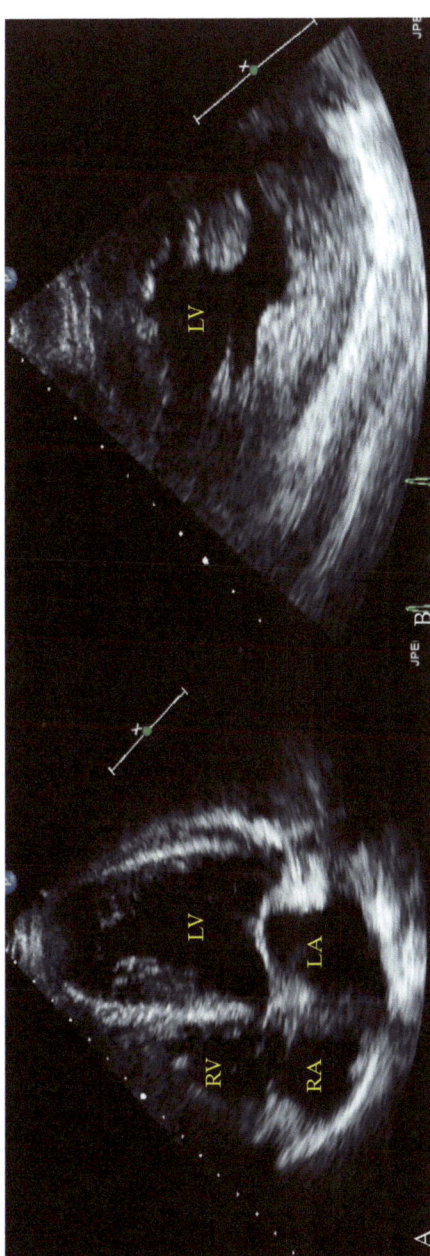

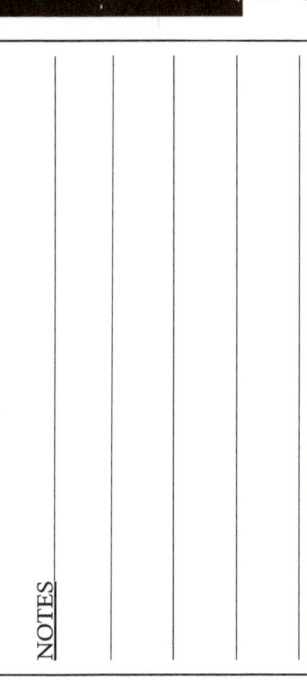

Fig. 24 Echo images showing LVH **A,** An apical 4-chamber view showing septal thickening. **B,** A parasternal short axis view showing concentric thickening of the LV wall.

NOTES

Case 21: A 54 y.o. man with NICM (EF 24%) presents in acute-on-chronic renal failure

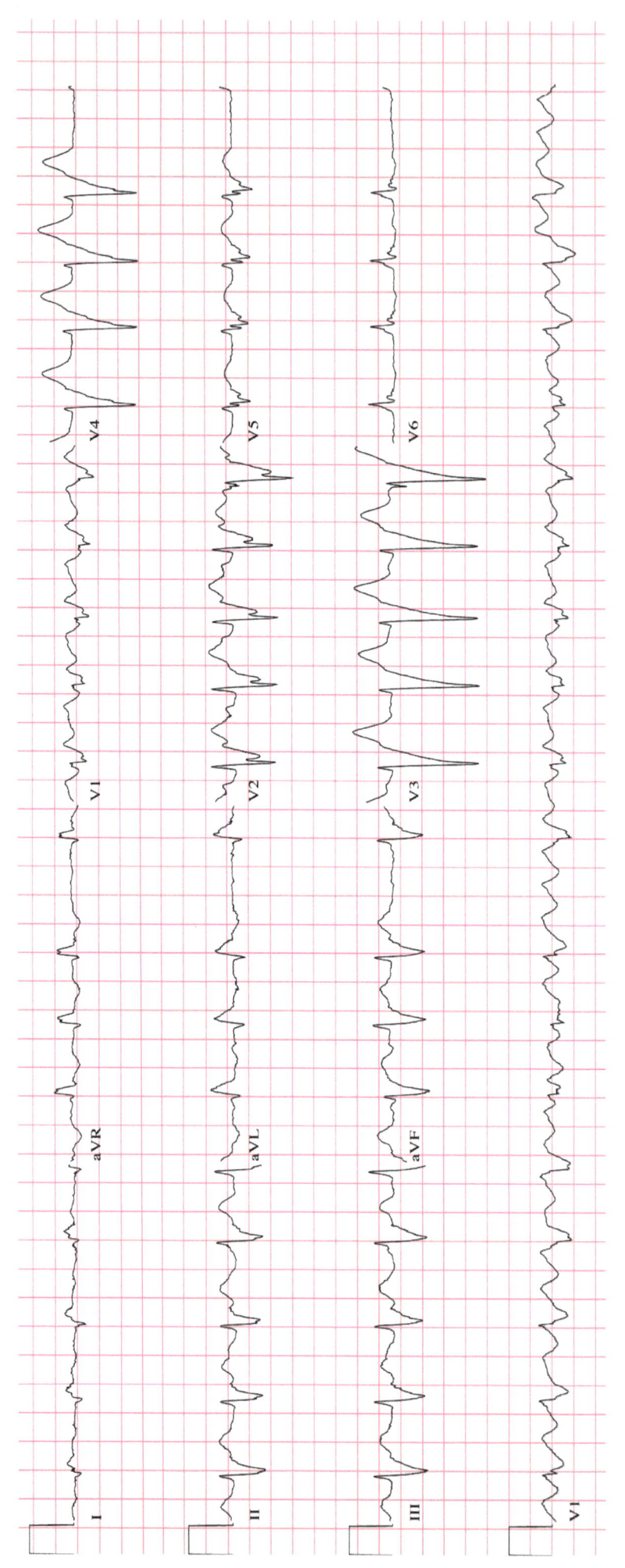

Hyperkalemia

Features:

- Tenting of T-waves- seen here in V_3-V_4
- Widened QRS > 120ms
- Downsloping STE- seen here best in V_3-V_4
- Widened, low amplitude or no P-wave [48,81]

Other findings in this case:

- Atrial fibrillation

Clinical Pearl:

- Widening QRS complex can merge with T-wave and form a classic sine wave pattern, which can result in asystole and VF [29,73]

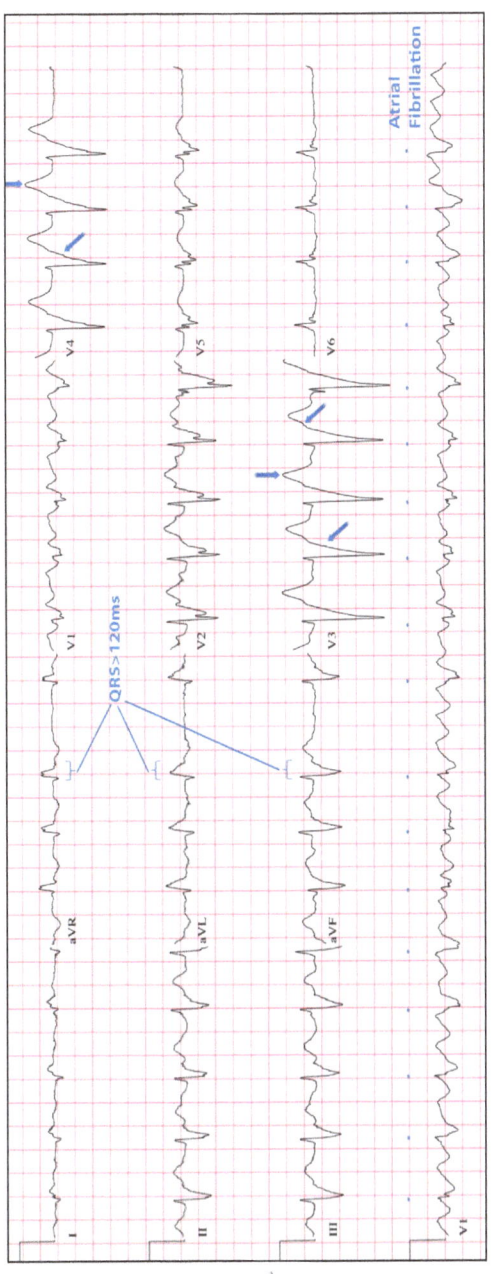

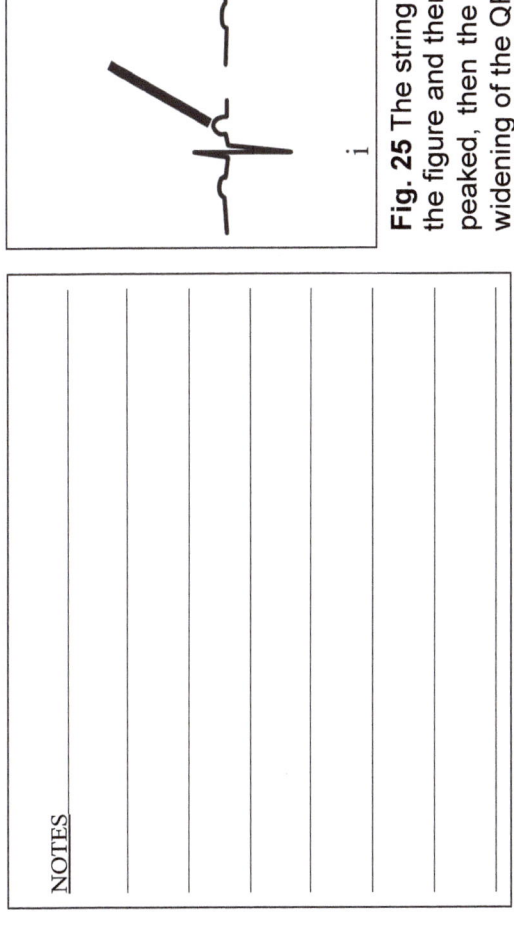

Fig. 25 The string theory of hyperkalemia. Imagine attaching a string to the T-wave as shown in the figure and then pulling in the direction of the black arrow. First the T-waves become tall and peaked, then the PR-segment widens and depresses with eventual loss of the P-wave and widening of the QRS which further devolves into a sine wave followed by asystole.

NOTES

Case 22: A 26 y.o. man with h/o VT

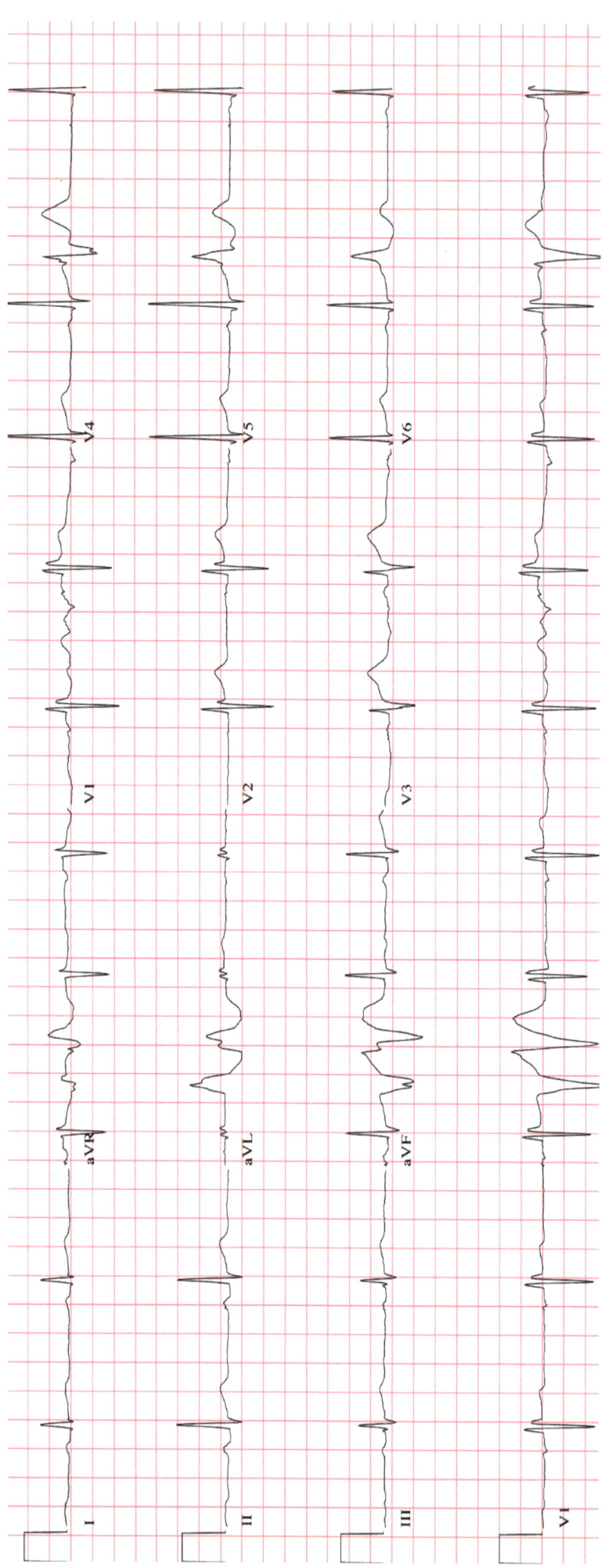

Brugada Syndrome

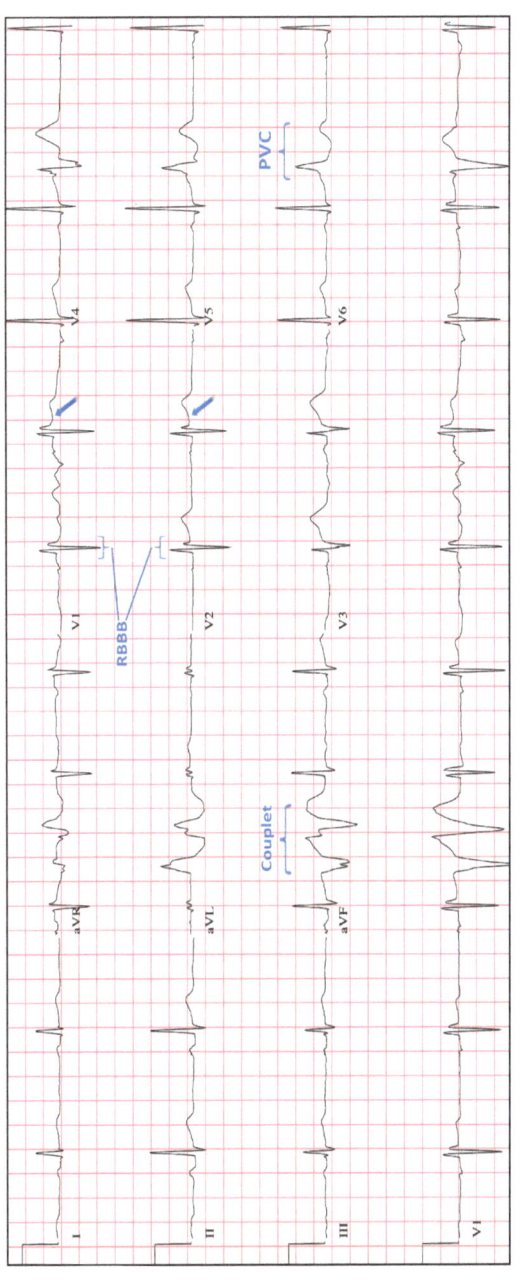

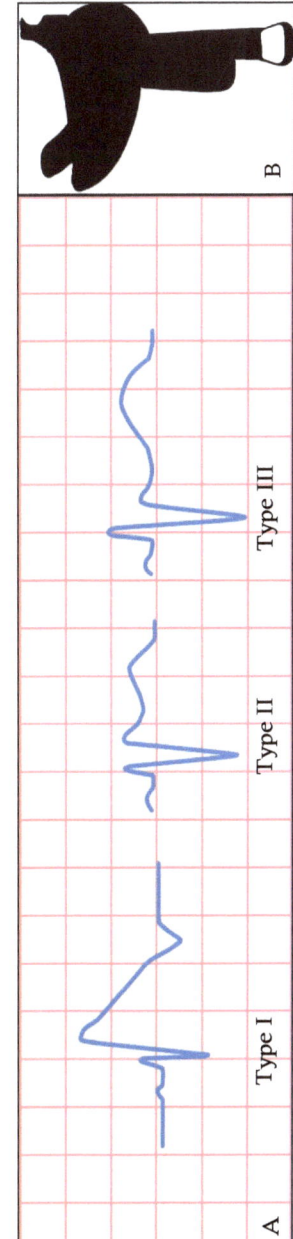

Features:

- Type 1- Coved STE >2mm or .2 mV in V_1-V_3 followed by a negative T wave with little or no isoelectric isolation (Brugada sign)[30,31,82] (Figure A)

- Type 2- High takeoff STE descending from J-wave in V_1-V_3 followed by positive or biphasic T-wave (saddleback configuration)[30,31,82]

- Type 3 (seen in this case)- Less than 1 mm of STE of either the coved type, saddle back type, or both[30,31,82]

- RSR' pattern in V_1 and V_2 indicates RBBB, which is frequently seen in Brugada Syndrome[30,31,82]

Clinical Pearl:

- R on T phenomena - PVCs occurring around the middle of the T-wave ("the vulnerable period") can induce VT. Note couplet in this example

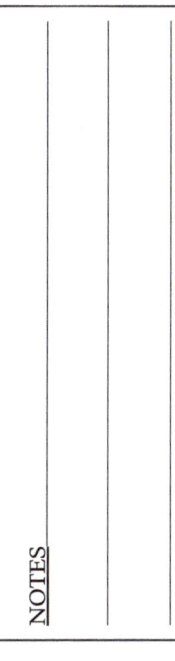

Fig. 26 A, Brugada Type I, II and III. **B**, Saddleback shape. Imagine the upper outline superimposed on the EKG in types II and III

NOTES

63

Case 23: A 27 y.o. man c/o acute onset dizziness a/w nausea

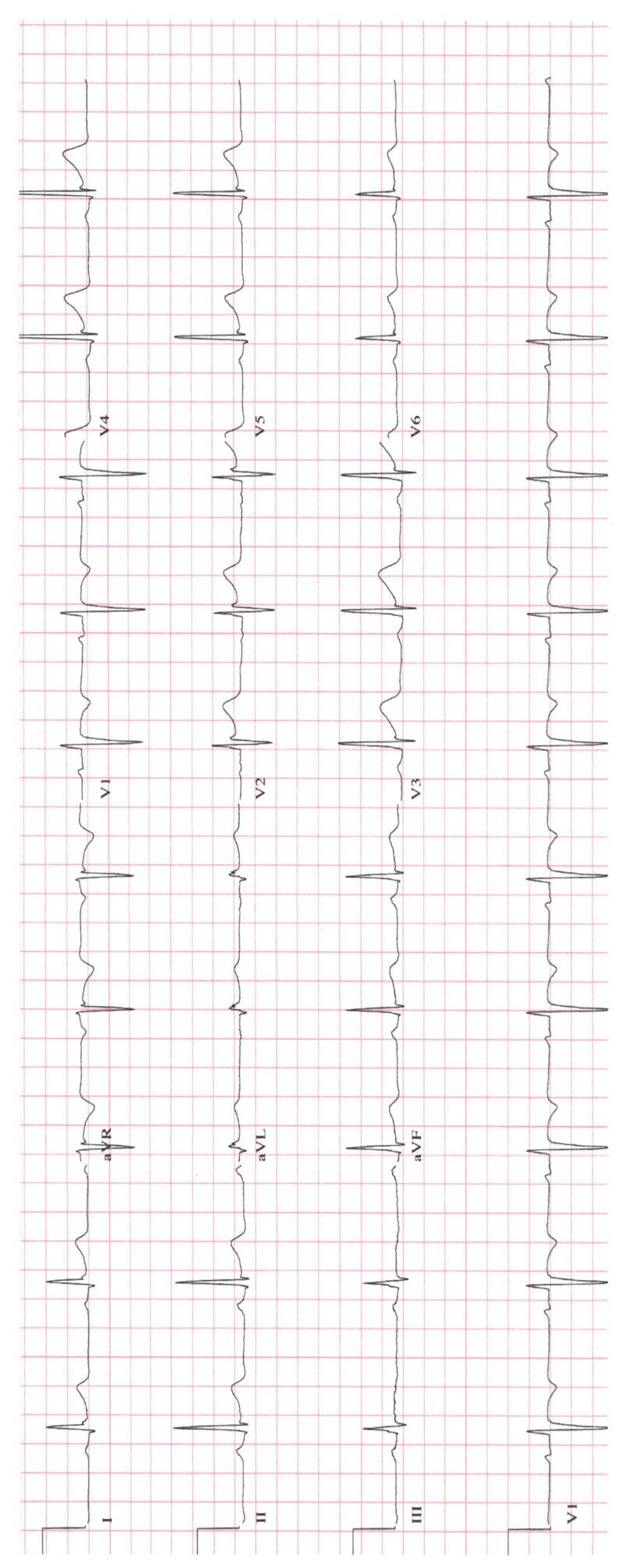

Early Repolarization

Features:
- Concave STE in V_3-V_6
- Compare the shape of these ST-segments to those in classic anterior MI (cases 2 & 3)
- Slurred terminal QRS complex
- J point notching in $V_3 - V_6$ [25,26,83-86]

Clinical Pearl:
- This is a benign condition seen most commonly in young, healthy, athletic males and african americans [25,26,83-86]

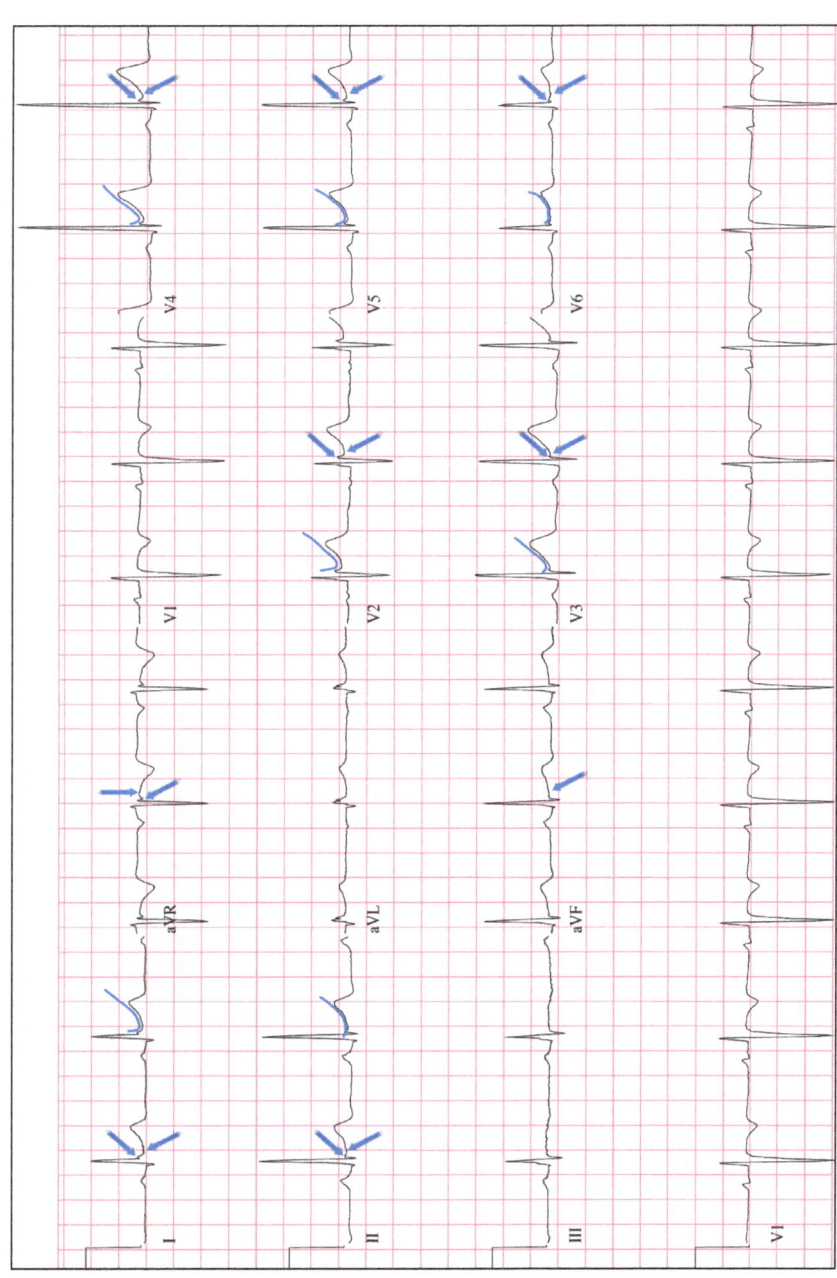

NOTES

Case 24: A 55 y.o. woman with HTN presents with a stroke and normal coronaries

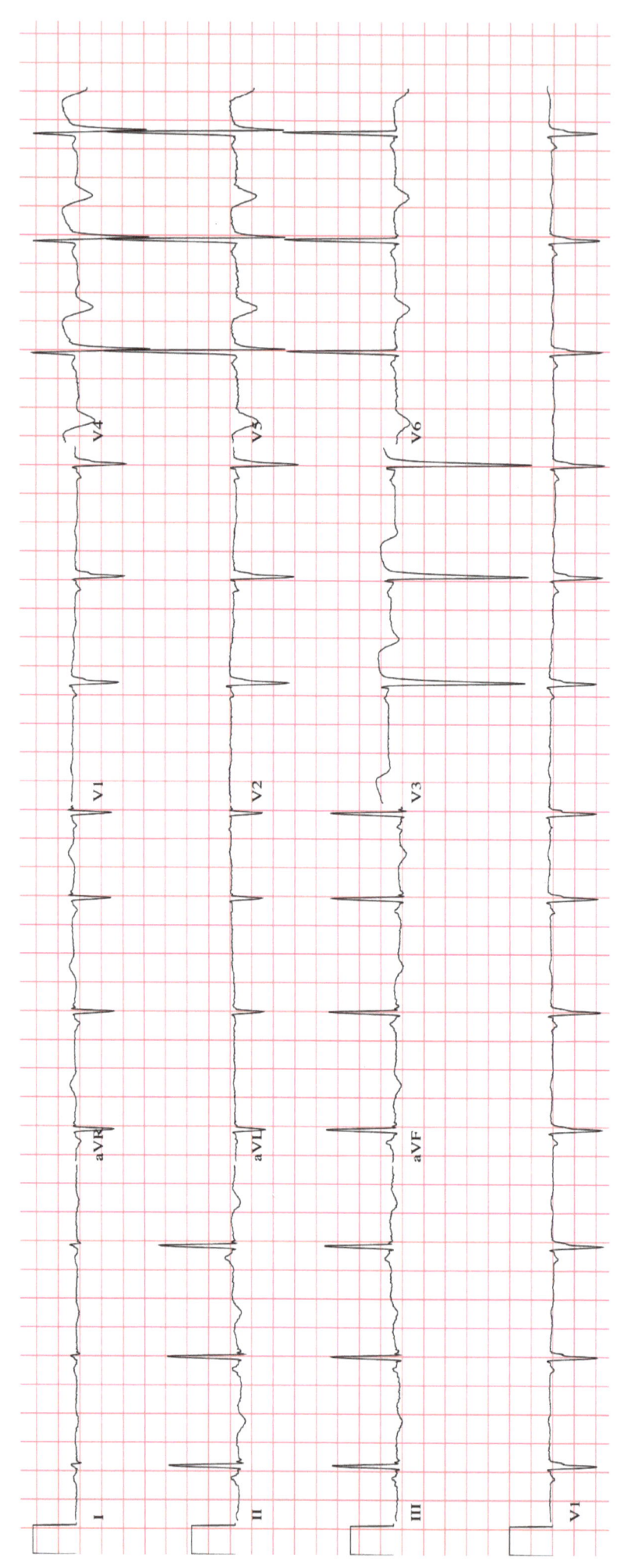

Takotsubo Cardiomyopathy

Features:

- Coronary angiography is usually performed to distinguish STEMI from Takotsubo cardiomyopathy.

- Acute phase
  - $\Sigma STE\ V_4–V_6/\Sigma STE\ V_1–V_3 \geq/=1$ + absence of reciprocal changes or abnormal Q waves can help to distinguish TC from an anterior MI with high sensitivity and specificity [87]

Other Findings:

- Note clot in LV apex (Figure A)

Clinical Pearl:

- The classic Takotsubo patient is a post-menopausal woman with severe emotional or other physiologic stress [37,87]
- Normal coronary arteries on angiography.
- Left ventricular dysfunction normalizes within several months.
- It is also known as Broken Heart Syndrome

<u>NOTES</u>

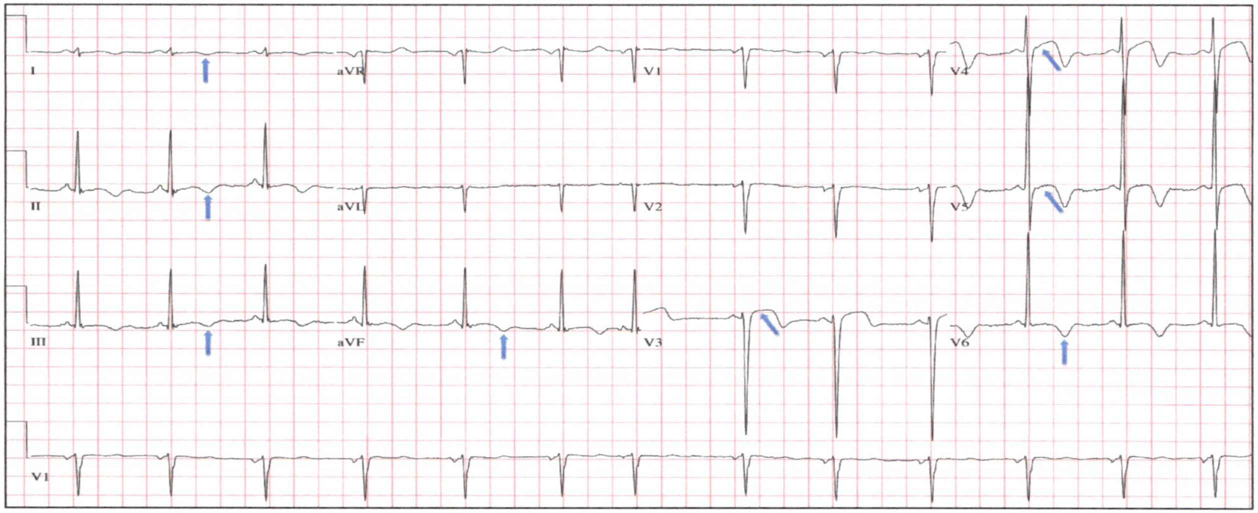

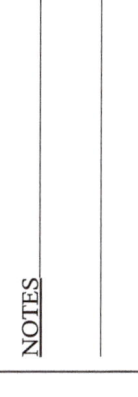

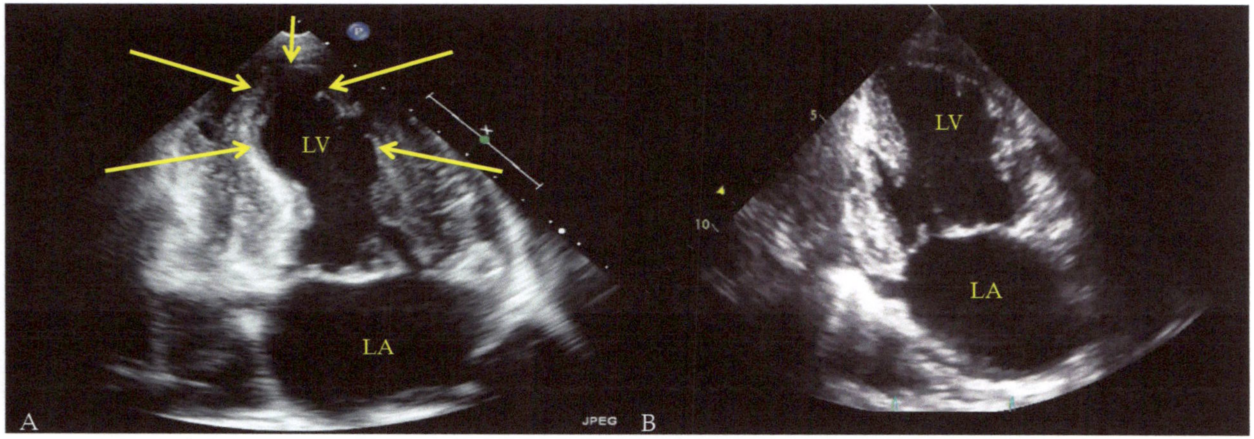

Fig. 27 Echocardiographic images showing LVH **A,** LV apical ballooning with clot (arrow). **B,** Repeat imaging showing resolution of apical aneurysm and clot.

INDEX

References

1. Wagner, G. S., MacFarlane, P., Wellens, H., Josephson, M., Gorgels, A., Mirvis, D. M., et al. (2009). AHA / ACCF / HRS recommendations for the standardization and interpretation of the electrocardiogram: Part VI: Acute ischemia/infarction: A scientific statement from the american heart association electrocardiography and arrhythmias committee, council on clinical cardiology; the american college of cardiology foundation; and the heart rhythm society. *Circulation, 119*(10), e262-e270.

2. Bradley, E. H., Herrin, J., Wang, Y., Barton, B. A., Webster, T. R., Mattera, J. A., et al. (2006). Strategies for reducing the door-to-balloon time in acute myocardial infarction. *New England Journal of Medicine, 355*(22), 2308-2320.

3. Rokos, I. C., French, W. J., Koenig, W. J., Stratton, S. J., Nighswonger, B., Strunk, B., et al. (2009). Integration of pre-hospital electrocardiograms and ST-elevation myocardial infarction receiving center (SRC) networks. impact on door-to-balloon times across 10 independent regions. *JACC: Cardiovascular Interventions, 2*(4), 339-346.

4. Rokos, I. C., French, W. J., Mattu, A., Nichol, G., Farkouh, M. E., Reiffel, J., et al. (2010). Appropriate cardiac cath lab activation: Optimizing electrocardiogram interpretation and clinical decision-making for acute ST-elevation myocardial infarction. *American Heart Journal, 160*(6), 995-1003.e8.

5. Rokos, I. C., Larson, D. M., Henry, T. D., Koenig, W. J., Eckstein, M., French, W. J., et al. (2006). Rationale for establishing regional ST-elevation myocardial infarction receiving center (SRC) networks. *American Heart Journal, 152*(4), 661-667.

6. Kontos, M. C., Kurz, M. C., Roberts, C. S., Joyner, S. E., Kreisa, L., Ornato, J. P., et al. (2010). An evaluation of the accuracy of emergency physician activation of the cardiac catheterization laboratory for patients with suspected ST-segment elevation myocardial infarction. *Annals of Emergency Medicine, 55*(5), 423-430.

7. Lau, J., Ioannidis, J. P. A., Balk, E. M., Milch, C., Terrin, N., Chew, P. W., et al. (2001). Diagnosing acute cardiac ischemia in the emergency department: A systematic review of the accuracy and clinical effect of current technologies. *Annals of Emergency Medicine, 37*(5), 453-460.

8. Swan, P. Y., Nighswonger, B., Boswell, G. L., & Stratton, S. J. (2009). Factors associated with false-positive emergency medical services triage for percutaneous coronary intervention. *Western Journal of Emergency Medicine, 10*(4), 208-212.

9. Mant, J., McManus, R. J., Oakes, R. A. L., Delaney, B. C., Barton, P. M., Deeks, J. J., et al. (2004). Systematic review and modeling of the investigation of acute and chronic chest pain presenting in primary care. *Health Technology Assessment, 8*(2), iii-78.

10. Engelen, D. J., Gorgels, A. P., Cheriex, E. C., De Muinck, E. D., Oude Ophuis, A. J., Dassen, W. R., et al. (1999). Value of the electrocardiogram in localizing the occlusion site in the left anterior descending coronary artery in acute anterior myocardial infarction. *Journal of the American College of Cardiology, 34*(2), 389-395.

11. Herz, I., Assali, A. R., Adler, Y., Solodky, A., & Sclarovsky, S. (1997). New electrocardiographic criteria for predicting either the right or left circumflex artery as the culprit coronary artery in inferior wall acute myocardial infarction. *American Journal of Cardiology, 80*(10), 1343-1345.

12. Zimetbaum, P. J., Krishnan, S., Gold, A., Carrozza II, J. P., & Josephson, M. E. (1998). Usefulness of ST-segment elevation in lead III exceeding that of lead II for identifying the location of the totally occluded coronary artery in inferior wall myocardial infarction. *American Journal of Cardiology, 81*(7), 918-919.

13. Huey, B. L., Beller, G. A., Kaiser, D. L., & Gibson, R. S. (1988). A comprehensive analysis of myocardial infarction due to left circumflex artery occlusion: Comparison with infarction due to right coronary artery and left anterior descending artery occlusion. *Journal of the American College of Cardiology, 12*(5), 1156-1166.

14. Indications for fibrinolytic therapy in suspected acute myocardial infarction: Collaborative overview of early mortality and major morbidity results from all randomised

trials of more than 1000 patients.(1994). Fibrinolytic Therapy Trialists' (FTT) Collaborative Group. *The Lancet, 343*(8893), 311-322.

15. Kontos, M. C., McQueen, R. H., Jesse, R. L., Tatum, J. L., & Ornato, J. P. (2001). Can myocardial infarction be rapidly identified in emergency department patients who have left bundle-branch block? *Annals of Emergency Medicine, 37*(5), 431-438.

16. Sgarbossa, E. B., Pinski, S. L., Barbagelata, A., Underwood, D. A., Gates, K. B., Topol, E. J., et al. (1996). Electrocardiographic diagnosis of evolving acute myocardial infarction in the presence of left bundle-branch block. *New England Journal of Medicine, 334*(8), 481-487.

17. Tabas, J. A., Rodriguez, R. M., Seligman, H. K., & Goldschlager, N. F. (2008). Electrocardiographic criteria for detecting acute myocardial infarction in patients with left bundle branch block: A meta-analysis. *Annals of Emergency Medicine, 52*(4), 329-336.e1.

18. Fesmire, F. M., Brady, W. J., Hahn, S., Decker, W. W., Diercks, D. B., Ghaemmaghami, C. A., et al. (2006). Clinical policy: Indications for reperfusion therapy in emergency department patients with suspected acute myocardial infarction. *Annals of Emergency Medicine, 48*(4), 358-383.

19. Zoghbi, G. J., Misra, V. K., Brott, B. C., Papapietro, S. E., Dai, D., Ou, F., et al. (2010). St elevation myocardial infarction due to left main culprit lesions: Percutaneous coronary intervention outcomes. *Journal of the American College of Cardiology, 55*(10s1), A183.E1712-A183.E1712.

20. Rostoff, P., Piwowarska, W., Gackowski, A., Konduracka, E., El Massri, N., Latacz, P., et al. (2007). Electrocardiographic prediction of acute left main coronary artery occlusion. *American Journal of Emergency Medicine, 25*(7), 852-855.

21. Smith, S. W., & Whitwam, W. (2006). Acute coronary syndromes. *Emergency Medicine Clinics of North America, 24*(1), 53-89.

22. Nikus, K., Pahlm, O., Wagner, G., Birnbaum, Y., Cinca, J., Clemmensen, P., et al. (2010). Electrocardiographic classification of acute coronary syndromes: A review by a committee of the international society for holter and non-invasive electrocardiology. *Journal of Electrocardiology, 43*(2), 91-103.

23. De Zwaan, C., Bar, F. W. H. M., & Wellens, H. J. J. (1982). Characteristic electrocardiographic pattern indicating a critical stenosis high in left anterior descending coronary artery in patients admitted because of impending myocardial infarction. *American Heart Journal, 103*(4 II), 730-736.

24. Collins, M. S., Carter, J. E., Dougherty, J. M., Majercik, S. M., Hodsden, J. E., & Logue, E. E. (1990). Hyperacute T-wave criteria using computer ECG analysis. *Annals of Emergency Medicine, 19*(2), 114-120.

25. Hiss, R. G., Lamb, L. E., & Allen, M. F. (1960). Electrocardiographic findings in 67,375 asymptomatic subjects. X. normal values*. *The American Journal of Cardiology, 6*(1), 200-231.

26. Surawicz, B., & Parikh, S. R. (2002). Prevalence of male and female patterns of early ventricular repolarization in the normal ECG of males and females from childhood to old age. *Journal of the American College of Cardiology, 40*(10), 1870-1876.

27. Ginzton, L. E., & Laks, M. M. (1982). The differential diagnosis of acute pericarditis from the normal variant: New electrocardiographic criteria. *Circulation, 65*(5), 1004-1009.

28. Levine, H.D., Wanzer, S.H., & Merrill, J.P. (1956). Dialyzable currents of injury in potassium intoxication resembling acute myocardial infarction or pericarditis. *Circulation, 13*(1), 29-36.

29. Montague, B. T., Ouellette, J. R., & Buller, G. K. (2008). Retrospective review of the frequency of ECG changes in hyperkalemia. *Clinical Journal of the American Society of Nephrology, 3*(2), 324-330.

30. Wilde, A. A. M., Antzelevitch, C., Borggrefe, M., Brugada, J., Brugada, R., Brugada, P., et al. (2002). Proposed diagnostic criteria for the brugada syndrome: Consensus report. *Circulation, 106*(19), 2514-2519.

31. Brugada, P., & Brugada, J. (1992). Right bundle branch block, persistent ST segment

elevation and sudden cardiac death: A distinct clinical and electrocardiographic syndrome. A multicenter report. *Journal of the American College of Cardiology, 20*(6), 1391-1396.

32. Sokolow, M., & Lyon, T. P. (1949). The ventricular complex in left ventricular hypertrophy as obtained by unipolar precordial and limb leads. *American Heart Journal, 37*(2), 161-186.

33. Levy, D., Labib, S. B., Anderson, K. M., Christiansen, J. C., Kannel, W. B., & Castelli, W. P. (1990). Determinants of sensitivity and specificity of electrocardiographic criteria for left ventricular hypertrophy. *Circulation, 81*(3), 815-820.

34. Shipley, R. A., & Hallaran, W. R. (1936). The four-lead electrocardiogram in two hundred normal men and women. *American Heart Journal, 11*(3), 325-345.

35. Geibel, A., Zehender, M., Kasper, W., Olschewski, M., Klima, C., & Konstantinides, S. V. (2005). Prognostic value of the ECG on admission in patients with acute major pulmonary embolism. *European Respiratory Journal, 25*(5), 843-848.

36. Sreeram, N., Cheriex, E. C., Smeets, J. L. R. M., Gorgels, A. P., & Wellens, H. J. J. (1994). Value of the 12-lead electrocardiogram at hospital admission in the diagnosis of pulmonary embolism. *American Journal of Cardiology, 73*(4), 298-303.

37. Inoue, M., Shimizu, M., Ino, H., Yamaguchi, M., Terai, H., Fujino, N., et al. (2005). Differentiation between patients with takotsubo cardiomyopathy and those with anterior acute myocardial infarction. *Circulation Journal, 69*(1), 89-94.

38. Sgarbossa, E. B., Birnbaum, Y., & Parrillo, J. E. (2001). Electrocardiographic diagnosis of acute myocardial infarction: Current concepts for the clinician. *American Heart Journal, 141*(4), 507-517.

39. Zimetbaum, P. J., & Josephson, M. E. (2003). Use of the electrocardiogram in acute myocardial infarction. *New England Journal of Medicine, 348*(10), 933-940.

40. Selwyn, A. P., Fox, K., Welman, E., & Shillingford, J. P. (1978). Natural history and evaluation of Q waves during acute myocardial infarction. *British Heart Journal, 40*(4), 383-387.

41. Birnbaum, Y., Sclarovsky, S., Solodky, A., Tschori, J., Herz, I., Sulkes, J., et al. (1993). Prediction of the level of left anterior descending coronary artery obstruction during anterior wall acute myocardial infarction by the admission electrocardiogram. *American Journal of Cardiology, 72*(11), 823-826.

42. Atar, S., Barbagelata, A., & Birnbaum, Y. (2006). Electrocardiographic diagnosis of ST-elevation myocardial infarction. *Cardiology Clinics, 24*(3), 343-365.

43. Aldrich, H. R., Wagner, N. B., Boswick, J., Corsa, A. T., Jones, M. G., Grande, P., . . . Wagner, G. S. (1988). Use of initial ST-segment deviation for prediction of final electrocardiographic size of acute myocardial infarcts. American Journal of Cardiology. Apr 1;61(10):749-53.

44. Wellens, H. J. J., Gorgels, Anton P. M., Doevendans,Pieter A.,. (2002). The ECG in acute myocardial infarction and unstable angina diagnosis and risk stratification. Springer, Boston, MA. 2002.

45. Tamura, A., Kataoka, H., Nagase, K., Mikuriya, Y., & Nasu, M. (1995). Clinical significance of inferior ST elevation during acute anterior myocardial infarction. *British Heart Journal, 74*(6), 611-614.

46. Sadanandan, S., Hochman, J. S., Kolodziej, A., Criger, D. A., Ross, A., Selvester, R., et al. (2003). Clinical and angiographic characteristics of patients with combined anterior and inferior ST-segment elevation on the initial electrocardiogram during acute myocardial infarction. *American Heart Journal, 146*(4), 653-661.

47. Yamaji, H., Iwasaki, K., Kusachi, S., Murakami, T., Hirami, R., Hamamoto, H., et al. (2001). Prediction of acute left main coronary artery obstruction by 12-lead electrocardiography: ST segment elevation in lead aVR with less ST segment elevation in lead V1. *Journal of the American College of Cardiology, 38*(5), 1348-1354.

48. Surawicz, B., & Knilans, T. K. (2008). *Chou's electrocardiography in clinical practice: Adult and pediatric.* Saunders/Elsevier. Philadelphia, PA.

49. Birnbaum, Y., Mahaffey, K. W., Criger, D. A., Gates, K. B., Barbash, G. I., Barbagelata, A., . . . Wagner, G. S. (2002). Grade III ischemia on presentation with acute myocardial infarction predicts rapid progression of necrosis and less myocardial salvage with thrombolysis. *Cardiology, 97*(3), 166-174.

50. Nielsen, B. L. (1973). ST segment elevation in acute myocardial infarction: Prognostic importance. *Circulation, 48*(2), 338-345.

51. Bonow, Robert O.,,Braunwald, Eugene,,. (2012). *Heart disease : A textbook of cardiovascular medicine*. Philadelphia, PA. Elsevier/Saunders.

52. Udall, J. A., & Ellestad, M. H. (1977). Predictive implications of ventricular premature contractions associated with treadmill stress testing. *Circulation, 56*(6), 985-989.

53. Verouden, N. J., Barwari, K., Koch, K. T., Henriques, J. P., Baan, J., Van Der Schaaf, R. J., et al. (2009). Distinguishing the right coronary artery from the left circumflex coronary artery as the infarct-related artery in patients undergoing primary percutaneous coronary intervention for acute inferior myocardial infarction. *Europace, 11*(11), 1517-1521.

54. Birnbaum, Y., Wagner, G. S., Barbash, G. I., Gates, K., Criger, D. A., Sclarovsky, S., et al. (1999). Correlation of angiographic findings and right (V1 to V3) versus left (V4 to V6) precordial ST-segment depression in inferior wall acute myocardial infarction. *American Journal of Cardiology, 83*(2), 143-148.

55. Sugiura, T., Iwasaka, T., Takehana, K., Nagahama, Y., Hasegawa, T., & Inada, M. (1993). *Precordial ST segment depression in patients with Q wave inferior myocardial infarction: Role of infarction-associated pericarditis.* American Heart Journal. Mar;125(3):672-5.

56. Wong, C. -., Freedman, S. B., Bautovich, G., Bailey, B. P., Bernstein, L., & Kelly, D. T. (1993). Mechanism and significance of precordial ST-segment depression during inferior wall acute myocardial infarction associated with severe narrowing of the dominant right coronary artery. *American Journal of Cardiology, 71*(12), 1025-1030.

57. Casas, R. E., Marriott, H. J. L., & Glancy, D. L. (1997). Value of leads V7–V9 in diagnosing posterior wall acute myocardial infarction and other causes of tall R waves in V1–V2. *The American Journal of Cardiology, 80*(4), 508-509.

58. Wei, J. Y., Markis, J. E., Malagold, M., & Braunwald, E. (1983). Cardiovascular reflexes stimulated by reperfusion of ischemic myocardium in acute myocardial infarction. *Circulation, 67*(4), 796-801.

59. Imazio M, Brucato A, Cemin R et al. A Randomized Trial of Colchicine for Acute Pericarditis. N Engl J Med 2013; 369: 1522-1528.

60. Menown, I. B. A., & Adgey, A. A. J. (2000). Improving the ECG classification of inferior and lateral myocardial infarction by inversion of lead aVR. *Heart, 83*(6), 657-660.

61. Willems, J. L., Robles De Medina, E. O., Bernard, R., Coumel, P., Fisch, C., Krikler, D., et al. (1985). Criteria for intraventricular conduction disturbances and pre-excitation. *Journal of the American College of Cardiology, 5*(6), 1261-1275.

62. Al-Faleh, H., Fu, Y., Wagner, G., Goodman, S., Sgarbossa, E., Granger, C., et al. (2006). Unraveling the spectrum of left bundle branch block in acute myocardial infarction: Insights from the assessment of the safety and efficacy of a new thrombolytic (ASSENT 2 and 3) trials. *American Heart Journal, 151*(1), 10-15.

63. Lopes, R. D., Siha, H., Fu, Y., Mehta, R. H., Patel, M. R., Armstrong, P. W., et al. (2011). Diagnosing acute myocardial infarction in patients with left bundle branch block. *American Journal of Cardiology, 108*(6), 782-788.

64. Somers, M. P., Brady, W. J., Perron, A. D., & Mattu, A. (2002). The prominant T wave: Electrocardiographic differential diagnosis. *The American Journal of Emergency Medicine, 20*(3), 243-251.

65. De Zwaan, C., Bar, F. W. H. M., & Wellens, H. J. J. (1982). Characteristic electrocardiographic pattern indicating a critical stenosis high in left anterior descending coronary artery in patients admitted because of impending myocardial

infarction. *American Heart Journal, 103*(4 II), 730-736.

66. Rhinehardt, J., Brady, W. J., Perron, A. D., & Mattu, A. (2002). Electrocardiographic manifestations of wellens' syndrome. *American Journal of Emergency Medicine, 20*(7), 638-643.

67. Vanpee, D., Courouble, P., Marchandise, B., Gillet, J. -., Tandy, T. K., & Bottomy, D. P. (1999). Wellens' syndrome [2] (multiple letters). *Annals of Emergency Medicine, 34*(5), 684-685.

68. Collins, M. S., Carter, J. E., Dougherty, J. M., Majercik, S. M., Hodsden, J. E., & Logue, E. E. (1990). Hyperacute T-wave criteria using computer ECG analysis. *Annals of Emergency Medicine, 19*(2), 114-120.

69. De Winter, R. J., Verouden, N. J. W., Wellens, H. J. J., & Wilde, A. A. M. (2008). A new ECG sign of proximal LAD occlusion. *New England Journal of Medicine, 359*(19), 2071-2073.

70. Surawicz, B., Childers, R., Deal, B. J., & Gettes, L. S. (2009). AHA/ACCF/HRS recommendations for the standardization and interpretation of the electrocardiogram: Part III: Intraventricular conduction disturbances: A scientific statement from the american heart association electrocardiography and arrhythmias committee, council on clinical cardiology; the american college of cardiology foundation; and the heart rhythm society. *Circulation, 119*(10), e235-e240.

71. Spodick, D. H. (1973). Diagnostic electrocardiographic sequences in acute pericarditis. significance of PR segment and PR vector changes. *Circulation, 48*(3), 575-580.

72. Surawicz, B., & Lasseter, K. C. (1970). Electrocardiogram in pericarditis. *The American Journal of Cardiology, 26*(5), 471-474.

73. Wang, K., Asinger, R. W., & Marriott, H. J. L. (2003). ST-segment elevation in conditions other than acute myocardial infarction. *New England Journal of Medicine, 349*(22), 2128-2135.

74. Spodick, D. H. (2003). Acute pericarditis: Current concepts and practice. *Journal of the American Medical Association, 289*(9), 1150-1153.

75. Bar, F. W., Brugada, P., Dassen, W. R., van der Werf, T., & Wellens, H. J. (1984). Prognostic value of Q waves, R/S ratio, loss of R wave voltage, ST-T segment abnormalities, electrical axis, low voltage and notching: Correlation of electrocardiogram and left ventriculogram. *Journal of the American College of Cardiology, 4*(1), 17-27.

76. Miller, R. R., Amsterdam, E. A., Bogren, H. G., Massumi, R. A., Zelis, R., & Mason, D. T. (1974). Electrocardiographic and cineangiographic correlations in assessment of the location, nature and extent of abnormal left ventricular segmental contraction in coronary artery disease. *Circulation, 49*(3), 447-454.

77. Ferrari, E., Imbert, A., Chevalier, T., Mihoubi, A., Morand, P., & Baudouy, M. (1997). The ECG in pulmonary embolism: Predictive value of negative T waves in precordial leads - 80 case reports. *Chest, 111*(3), 537-543.

78. Jimenez, D., & Konstantinides, S. (2005). ECG for risk stratification in patients with pulmonary embolism (multiple letters) [7]. *European Respiratory Journal, 26*(2), 366-367.

79. Casale, P. N., Devereux, R. B., Alonso, D. R., Campo, E., & Kligfield, P. (1987). Improved sex-specific criteria of left ventricular hypertrophy for clinical and computer interpretation of electrocardiograms: Validation with autopsy findings. *Circulation, 75*(3), 565-572.

80. Casale, P. N., Devereux, R. B., Kligfield, P., Eisenberg, R. R., Miller, D. H., Chaudhary, B. S., et al. (1985). Electrocardiographic detection of left ventricular hypertrophy: Development and prospective validation of improved criteria. *Journal of the American College of Cardiology, 6*(3), 572-580.

81. Surawicz, B. (1967). Relationship between electrocardiogram and electrolytes. *American Heart Journal, 73*(6), 814-834.

82. Brugada, J., & Brugada, P. (1997). Further characterization of the syndrome of right bundle branch block, ST segment elevation, and sudden cardiac death. *Journal of Cardiovascular Electrophysiology, 8*(3), 325-331.

83. Klatsky, A. L., Oehm, R., Cooper, R. A., Udaltsova, N., & Armstrong, M. A. (2003). The early repolarization normal variant electrocardiogram: Correlates and consequences. *American Journal of Medicine, 115*(3), 171-177.

84. Spodick, D. H. (1976). Differential characteristics of the electrocardiogram in early repolarization and acute pericarditis. *New England Journal of Medicine, 295*(10), 523-526.

85. Derval, N., Shah, A., & Jaïs, P. (2011). Definition of early repolarization: A tug of war. *Circulation, 124*(20), 2185-2186.

86. Mehta, M. C., & Jain, A. C. (1995). Early repolarization on scalar electrocardiogram. *American Journal of the Medical Sciences, 309*(6), 305-311.

87. Ogura, R., Hiasa, Y., Takahashi, T., Yamaguchi, K., Fujiwara, K., Ohara, Y., et al. (2003). *Specific findings of the standard 12-lead ECG in patients with 'takotsubo' cardiomyopathy: Comparison with the findings of acute anterior myocardial infarction.* Circulation Journal. Aug;67(8):687-90.